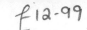
£12-99.

the BULLYING culture

culture

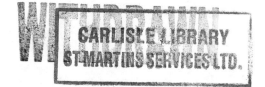
0750652012

The BULLYING culture

culture

cause · effect · harm reduction

Ruth Hadikin · Muriel O'Driscoll

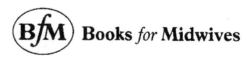 **Books** *for* **Midwives**

OXFORD AUCKLAND BOSTON JOHANNESBURG MELBOURNE NEW DELHI

Books for Midwives
An imprint of Butterworth-Heinemann
Linacre House, Jordan Hill, Oxford OX2 8DP
225 Wildwood Avenue, Woburn, MA 01801-2041
A division of Reed Educational and Professional Publishing Ltd

℞ A member of the Reed Elsevier plc group

First published 2000

© Ruth Hadikin and Muriel O'Driscoll 2000

British Library Cataloguing in Publication Data
A catalogue record for this book is available from the British Library

ISBN 0 7506 5201 2

Printed and Bound in Great Britain by
Biddles Ltd, Guildford and Kings Lynn

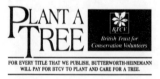

Contents

About the authors   vi

Introduction   1

Chapter 1   7
What is workplace bullying?

Chapter 2   29
Historical and sociological factors:
how the NHS bullying culture developed

Chapter 3   43
Why and how do bullies bully?

Chapter 4   75
The effects of bullying

Chapter 5   103
The boss, the bully and the law

Chapter 6   115
Acknowledging and altering a bullying
workplace: guidance for managers

Chapter 7   149
Learning the lessons:
the NHS as a developing organisation

Suggested further reading   169

Contacts and resources   170

References   172

Index   175

About the authors

Ruth Hadikin BScHons (1st class), Cert Ed, ADM, RM, RN, executive and business coach, author and public speaker.

Ruth, previously a community midwife, midwife teacher and steward for the Royal College of Midwives, now applies her wisdom and expertise in assisting her clients to achieve personal, business and professional development goals. Her clients include NHS managers and executives in addition to business clients, writers, public speakers and others. She provides workshops and teleconferences on many topics including coaching, workplace bullying, life planning and writing for publication. A member of the International Coach Federation and past chair of their communications committee, Ruth may be contacted by telephone on 01704 896039 or by e-mail at: RHAssocs@aol.com or visit her website at: http://www.ruthhadikin.com

Muriel O'Driscoll MA, RM, MTD, FPCerts, Psychosexual Dip, freelance educator, expert witness, counsellor and therapist.

Previously a Principal Lecturer in Midwifery, Muriel has carved out a niche for herself working with young people at the Wirral Brook Advisory Centre and as a teacher at Skelmersdale College. She also runs a successful business, Healthfirst, that encompasses psychosexual therapy and stress management, expert witness reports for midwifery and stress-related litigation and an education service. Muriel lectures extensively on these and other topics and has published many articles in a variety of professional journals. She may be contacted by telephone on 0151 928 0596 or by e-mail at: muriel@healthfirstconsultants.co.uk or visit her website at: http://www.healthfirstconsultants.co.uk/

Introduction

*[interpersonal] skills enable the midwife
to understand, interpret and communicate,
and so foster the development of a
midwife-client relationship that is caring,
nurturing and supportive.*

(O'Driscoll and Hadikin, 1997)

Unfortunately, as research now demonstrates, not all social interactions are positive experiences. As human beings we influence each other through our interactions. Where the experience is positive it has a positive psychological impact and conversely, where the experience is negative it has a negative psychological impact. Intimidating behaviour is an example of a negative social interaction. By definition it is behaviour which is intended to have a negative effect upon the recipient, namely to cause them to feel intimidated. Aggression, bullying, harassment and violence are examples of behaviours which intimidate and as such are included in this book. The authors, as midwives, have focused largely on the maternity services but the lessons to be learned should be heeded throughout the National Health Service (NHS). In the wake of the Allitt enquiry (Department of Health, 1994) everyone providing healthcare should be concerned about aggressive, bullying carers.

Most of us are aware that harassment can take place at work but are probably unaware of the full extent of this problem in a large, busy, organisation such as the NHS. In 1995 Ruth Hadikin was carrying out research for an article she was writing on morale in midwifery. She heard stories from midwives who, in effect, were being bullied at work (though the midwives did not describe their experiences in these terms). This led her to conduct telephone interviews with midwives to ask about their experiences and ascertain the context within which the bullying took place. Some of their experiences are included in this book as case studies, though the names given have been changed to protect confidentiality. As a Royal College of Midwives (RCM) steward, Hadikin had a network of contacts throughout the UK. Her findings were consistent, and nation-wide.

From her original survey, one worrying aspect appeared to be common in many of the midwives' stories. Despite working in NHS Trusts as geographically distant from one another as Newcastle and Cornwall, midwives, at that time, were suggesting that a callous (later known as 'bullying') management style was deliberately adopted by Midwifery Managers and condoned by senior NHS management for reasons which will be explained later in this book.

Rumours were rife among delegates at the RCM conference that same year, with whisperings of a widespread NHS 'witch-hunt' against 'G' grade midwives to force them into resignation or dismissal. To place this in perspective, at about the same time, similar reports had appeared in the national press: so these rumours could not have just been the invention of a few midwives with overactive imaginations. In July 1995 a report in The Guardian claimed that:

> *An increase in bullying at work has been partly caused by 'harsh' management practices*

and

> *...that employers tolerated bullying and some even encouraged a bullying management style.*

It was to be discovered that such reports were not entirely without foundation: The Guardian had taken its story from the Manufacturing, Science and Finance (MSF) union's report of their conference, held the preceding year (MSF, 1994).

Following her own preliminary findings, and having read the MSF report, Hadikin wrote to the RCM to enlist their help in identifying the extent of the problem in midwifery. She reported her initial findings to the RCM and suggested that the next step must be a quantitative survey to assess the prevalence of bullying among midwives in general. As a result she was invited to participate in the design of a questionnaire, 1000 of which were sent to a randomly selected cross-section of RCM members throughout the UK. The results are shocking (RCM, 1996) and should be of concern to everyone interested in the maternity services in particular, or the NHS in general.

The questionnaire was designed to assess not only how many midwives had been bullied, but who was doing the bullying. The results showed that 51% of respondents were bullied by a more senior colleague, 41% by a Midwifery Manager and 21% by a Supervisor of Midwives (RCM, 1996). Following this survey, Hadikin invited midwives who had experienced harassment, intimidation, or bullying to write to her, describing the experience in their own words. This formed the basis of her BSc dissertation (unpublished) which has been expanded to form the basis for this book. Rumours that 'G' grade staff were being 'singled out for special treatment' were not supported by this study; however this and other studies have since shown that a widespread culture of bullying permeates throughout the NHS. All NHS employees are at risk, either directly or indirectly (witnessing for example), of experiencing bullying behaviour at some stage during their NHS employment.

Concerned about the implications of this for midwifery care, the authors include stories not only from midwives, but from users of maternity services who have felt intimidated. We have included these stories as case studies because we felt it especially important to hear their own words: their descriptions of what happened and, perhaps more importantly, their understanding of what was happening. For this reason we wanted to hear from both midwives and women regardless of whether they described their experience as harassment, intimidation, bullying or violence. We were interested in the names women themselves used to describe and explain their experience. It is interesting to note that not a single male midwife contacted us about his experience. In the one letter we received from a man, he was adding to his wife's description of her experience. For this reason, and because the repeated use of 'he or she' can make for cumbersome reading, the female pronoun has been used throughout this book merely to facilitate reading and in no way is it intended to indicate sexism. There are gender issues around bullying however, which will be discussed in Chapter 3.

When a bullying culture is as deeply entrenched as it is in the NHS it is easy to assume that the situation is beyond repair. This is not the case. Any organisation can change the culture through effective development of staff and management. This does not mean attending a one-off study day and then forgetting all about it. This means a continuing programme of organisational development which includes everyone from ancillary staff to the Chief Executive, and consists of performance review, dealing with problem behaviour, coaching, mentoring and support structures. NHS Trust executives should recognise their limitations and call in outside agencies to facilitate organisational change on such an enormous scale.

Such culture shift is necessary to enable the introduction of 'jointism': collaborative employee relations which steer away from the confrontational 'us and them' industrial relations which have been the hallmark of NHS personnel management. Effective two-way communication is essential to promote trust, eradicate problem behaviour such as bullying and create a working environment that facilitates the growth and development of all staff.

The NHS can move towards becoming a healthy, learning organisation. Whilst the authors have focused on one issue, which they see as the major barrier to change within the NHS, this book offers solutions to how similar issues can be addressed jointly: by both management and staff-side organisations, without the old-style confrontationalism.

The language and style in this book takes account of the convergence of ideas and professional approaches which typifies modern management. It is designed to be 'readable' across all NHS professional groups. We have therefore reduced professional 'jargon' to a minimum. Where we have used midwifery terms we have offered an explanation for non-Midwifery Managers, and where we have used management jargon, we have offered an explanation for midwives. In this way we hope this book will be educational, as well as informative. The authors see such books as the future of jointism: where professional jargon is reduced, a common language is understood by all who are living and working within the NHS, and in this way we can begin to understand each other. Then staff employed in the NHS can move away from the 'us and them' siege mentality and move towards being 'we' together.

We do not include a separate discussion of racial harassment, sexual harassment and discrimination on the grounds of age, disability or sexual orientation in this book. Rather, due to the constraints of space, we hope that these issues are adequately incorporated into our discussions on how to handle 'problem behaviours' in general, in addition to bullying. Some of these will be referred to as we discuss relevant legislation, and we hope that our suggestions and advice to bullying victims can also be of help to those who identify themselves with one of these groups.

Chapter 1

What is workplace bullying?

Bullying is the aggressive behaviour arising from the deliberate intent to cause physical or psychological distress to others.

Randall, 1997

Workplace bullying has become an issue for many people working in the National Health Service (NHS) and the organisations which represent them. The *Nursing Times* has surveyed its readership and organised campaigns to tackle bullying, whilst staff organisations such as the Royal College of Nursing (RCN), the Manufacturing Science and Finance union (MSF) and the Royal College of Midwives (RCM) have taken steps such as organising seminars and campaigns or carrying out membership surveys. What, exactly, is workplace bullying? Is bullying in the NHS a problem, and is it an issue which should concern NHS managers?

Bullying: fact or fiction?

Why is there suddenly all this talk of workplace bullying? Is a new phenomenon taking hold in the British workplace or is this just another manifestation of the 'victim culture', with everyone being a victim these days, and no one accepting responsibility for what happens to them?

Managers are well aware of the fact that in large organisations, such as the NHS, interpersonal conflict is bound to occur and is part of everyday life. This has always been the case, especially where you have such a mixture of people from all walks of life working in one organisation. Some of the incidents which are reported to managers often appear so trivial that it can be hard to imagine that this should be taken seriously.

The problem for NHS managers is often how to decide whether this is a genuine concern or whether it is just part of a political storm whipped up by staff-side organisations in an attempt to gain cheap political points. If there is a real and tangible risk to the health and safety of staff, patients and the health of the organisation then it certainly is a matter of grave concern to NHS managers. So what is going on in the NHS?

Whilst it is true that conflict is not new, what is new is how we view it and its effects on the individuals concerned. Throughout the last ten years there has been a shift in management styles throughout the service industries towards Human Resource Management and a recognition that within large service-based industries, such as the health service, people are an organisation's prime asset. Within this context a healthy organisation is one based upon healthy assets... in this case people. Managers are now beginning to realise the advantages of the carrot over the stick.

One of the key areas targeted by the NHS human resources strategy launched in November 1998 is the level of sickness and absence in the NHS. Randall (1997) suggests that in any organisation where high sickness and absence levels cause problems workplace bullying should always be considered a possibility.

According to a survey carried out by the University of Stafford (cited by MSF, 1994), from a sample of 1137 men and women, 78 per cent had witnessed bullying whilst 51 per cent had experienced it themselves. The statistics on workplace bullying vary, with some reports claiming as many as 1 in 8 employees experience bullying whilst others claim 1 in 4. For example, the Royal College of Midwives (RCM, 1996) surveyed 1000 members and found that 43 per cent of respondents had experienced bullying and that 31 per cent of these were still being bullied.

The problem with research of this kind is that of definition. However, as managers, we must consider the impact of as much as 78 per cent of the workforce witnessing bullying behaviour. More extensive research is being undertaken by the University of Manchester Institute of Science and Technology (UMIST) under the supervision of Professor Cary Cooper which should shed some light on what exactly is happening in British workplaces, but until the results of this research are known it may be helpful to look at some background information which may illustrate some of the issues pertinent to the NHS.

In July 1995 a small item in *The Guardian* reported that:

An increase in bullying at work has been partly caused by "harsh" management practices

and

...that employers tolerated bullying and some even encouraged a bullying management style.

So what exactly do we mean by workplace bullying and can managers really be held responsible? Despite media sensationalism, the comments above may hold an element of truth, at least in some cases and with some managers. Unfortunately there has, in the past, been an element of respect for a bullying manager, one who 'keeps a tight ship' and manages by a reign of terror. It has long been a management myth that the authoritarian manager gets more done because his or her staff 'jump to it' and are too afraid to question orders. However it is now believed that the reverse is true: that this style of management stifles creativity and can impede performance.

It is difficult to address issues such as workplace bullying within an adversarial model of industrial relations. A genuine culture of two-way communication between staff and management within an organisation is essential if this problem is to be eradicated. This means listening as well as talking, on both sides.

Partly because of the move towards effective management of human resources, and the trend towards the application of psychology to organisational situations, there is increasing recognition of how confrontation, aggression, harassment and even violence can have a detrimental effect on performance by increasing stress to unacceptably, unhealthy, high levels. Confrontational in-house politics creates an environment which fosters aggressive behaviour.

It is also now being recognised that bullying is even more likely to occur where workplace stress is a factor to begin with. High stress workplaces are 'vulnerable' in that confrontation, or bullying behaviour, is more likely to occur in such areas.

... a hidden epidemic of intentional aggression... (Randall, 1997)

We have all felt humiliated or embarrassed at times. Sometimes a colleague can speak without thinking and may inadvertently hurt our feelings, so what is the difference between this and bullying or intimidation? The difference is one of intent, which makes it all the more difficult to discern, yet most of us are all too aware when we are being deliberately bullied or intimidated. Reports of bosses (ITV documentary Aug/Sept 1998) who walk into the office with a ready made 'dunce' hat which they force one of their employees to wear all afternoon can hardly be passed off as an unkind remark said in the heat of the moment, and go way beyond 'normal' office humour.

Part of the problem for managers is that there is separate legislation dealing with harassment, be it sexual or racial, or indeed whether it could be classed as stalking. Managers often find it hard to decide an appropriate route through which to deal with incidents because of the limitations of the organisation's policies and procedures. This confusion can lead to behaviour going unchecked until it becomes part of a department's, if not the organisation's, culture.

Definition

Unfortunately for managers there is no consensus definition of bullying. Ruth Lea, representing the Institute of Directors, claimed in a recent television documentary:

It's not bullying – it's not persistent.

This illustrates how easy it is for managers to confuse bullying with harassment. It also illustrates why bullying behaviour must be mentioned separately, and explicitly, in harassment policies. There are many behaviours which may not fit easily into a definition of harassment yet, if they cause psychological harm, the employee may still have a case to bring against an employer for a failure in their duty of care. It is therefore imperative that managers have a clear understanding of workplace bullying, and that organisations have an appropriate working definition of bullying behaviour. So what, then, constitutes an appropriate working definition?

Describing and labelling

To solve a problem you must first acknowledge that it exists, and to do this you must give it a name. Recognition is essential if bullying is to be legitimately challenged. In our survey some midwives remarked that such behaviour 'has always gone on in midwifery'. Is it so widespread that it is accepted and to a degree normalised? One of the authors remembers an incident, as a student, when a midwife slapped a woman's leg during labour. Was this an isolated case or typical of a bullying culture that we accept as 'normal'? In the NHS it is time each of us seriously examined our own attitude towards such behaviour.

Bullying in the medical profession is sometimes referred to in endearing terms as though it is acceptable if it is for our own good:

Dr. Jones is such a bully, he never allows me to skip this diet.

Have NHS staff gradually assimilated into this culture without recognising it? Where bullying exists it must be recognised and named as such.

The term 'bullying' is increasingly being used as an 'umbrella term', incorporating concepts such as harassment, intimidation, aggression and/or violence. Midwives do not often describe their experiences as bullying. The midwives interviewed in our survey tended to use terms such as aggression, intimidation, 'cold-heartedness' and harassment. The term bullying was used either when more than one person was being bullied, so the perpetrator was labelled as 'a bully', or when the incidents occurred over a prolonged period. This makes it difficult to assess whether the midwives involved had similar experiences if they were not all using the same language or indeed had no language or labels with which to describe their experiences. Comments such as:

> bullying has always gone on in midwifery

lead one to question what, precisely, has 'always gone on', how long such behaviour has been present and why it appears to go unchallenged?

Workplace bullying is therefore nothing new, but rather it is a term which attempts to define a phenomenon which can include aggression, intimidation, harassment and even violence. One of the difficulties of not having a label is that is becomes difficult for victims to understand what is happening to them. If a behaviour fits into a neat category such as a 'violent incident' or racial or sexual harassment, it is easier for us to recognise it for what it is, and understand how the victim feels, though it is still difficult behaviour to challenge. The problem is compounded when a victim is subject to low-level persistent harassment which feels very real to the victim, but which colleagues may not notice, or the perpetrator can laugh off and say 'it was only harmless fun!' (This, incidentally is no less real, and has been demonstrated to produce stress and aggressive behaviour in primates!) Such behaviour requires definition if we are to begin to recognise patterns and attempt to understand the dynamics of the interaction. This is only a first step towards tackling the problem, resolving the issues and making the NHS a dignified and emotionally safer environment in which to work.

Beginning academic research into this subject has led to attempts to arrive at a definition of the phenomenon. Though much of the research had, until recently, been carried out in Scandinavia (where workplace bullying is known as 'mobbing') there are now some definitions which are beginning to tackle the problem of what we in Britain mean by the term workplace bullying.

Definition is difficult in this subject which has only recently attracted the attention of academics. The Scandinavian term 'mobbing' is interesting because it has connotations of behaviour which we in Britain may not typically associate with the common use of the term bullying. In some of our case studies, which are illustrated throughout this book, we describe behaviour which, though it may not sound much like bullying to the reader, nevertheless is offensive behaviour which makes people feel uncomfortable in the workplace and could even be psychologically damaging.

Research is now increasingly being carried out on this subject and on the effects of bullying on the workplace and productivity. Contrary to popular managerial myths, the evidence so far suggests that a bully in the workplace actually disrupts working practices and decreases productivity. This is even more evident in service industries, where people and effective personnel management are so important.

The term bullying is therefore used to describe various behaviours which could psychologically harm the recipient. Rather than being side-tracked by various academic definitions, it would be wise for managers to focus on the effects on the victim; the legal concept of psychiatric harm; the employer's duty of care; and use these as the basis for a practical working definition. Once in the courtroom the judge is less likely to be interested in whether you call it bullying or harassment than whether the employer should have seen it coming and taken appropriate steps to protect their employee.

It may just be a matter of time before a consensus definition of bullying is reached. It would certainly make life simpler for policy makers. The Swedish term 'mobbing' encompasses a spectrum of aggressive and harassing behaviours which can occur in the workplace and which may harm an individual. Other commentators have coined the phrase 'psychological terrorism' in their attempts to seek an all-encompassing definition. The use of the term bullying in Britain can tend to make the whole subject appear more 'normal' due to the familiarity of the term and our familiarity with school yard bullying. This can lend the term a certain acceptability and sometimes trivialise the experience as though it is something that should be relegated to the school yard. This, in turn, can prevent people from complaining.

Any subsequent complaint could be seen as an expression of the victim's own inadequacies to cope with 'normal' employment interactions, which may bring about perceived loss of status or draw unwelcome attention to the individual. There is also the connotation with playground bullying of the past, where 'telltales' were despised by both children and teachers. These feelings, that it is unacceptable to tell tales or report when someone has upset you or hurt your feelings, are ingrained within many adults making a complaint about a bully very difficult. It can also resurrect the reaction of influential adults in a child's experience when they did complain:

Just ignore it and don't let them see that you're upset
Go and hit them back and don't come running to me!

The memories of these phrases add to the reluctance to report bullying.

By using terminology that makes the bullying behaviour an unacceptable practice, we elevate the complainant to the status of a hero, rather than a victim. In exploring some of the definitions which have been suggested in Britain it can be seen that the emphasis is on the effects on the individual, or victim. This is important to bear in mind when adopting a working definition, for the legal reasons mentioned above, because it is the victim that is most likely to suffer damage and hence bring a case against the employer.

The Guardian reported on a conference held by MSF (1994), which examined the issue of bullying at work. In her keynote speech at the conference, Andrea Adams gave the following definition of bullying:

We are talking here about the persistent demeaning and downgrading of human beings, through vicious words and cruel unseen acts which gradually undermine their confidence and self-esteem. It usually affects a number of staff at any one time, but through fear of further recriminations, if they speak out, it is typical for these people to remain silent. (MSF, 1994)

Following on from the conference in 1994, MSF produced a guide on workplace bullying which included the following definition:

> *persistent, offensive, abusive, intimidating, malicious or insulting behaviour, abuse of power or unfair penal sanctions, which makes the recipient feel upset, threatened, humiliated or vulnerable, which undermines their self-confidence and which may cause them to suffer stress* (Lyons, Tivey & Ball, 1995)

Though these definitions have since been widely used by staff-side organisations and individuals campaigning for change in employment legislation, we suggest that they are generally unhelpful to employers as a working definition because of the word 'persistent' which, as mentioned earlier, adds to the confusion that exists between bullying and harassment.

Of course harassment can be a form of bullying but an isolated incident can also be bullying. According to Randall (1997):

> *aggressive behaviour does not have to be regular or repeated for it to be bullying behaviour.*

The current trend towards defining bullying in terms of its effects on the victim, facilitates addressing the issue through legal frameworks (using the concept of psychiatric injury which will be discussed in Chapter 5) and enables disciplinary procedures to be developed and implemented against bullying behaviours in the workplace. For this reason we recommend that employers should adopt a working definition which focuses attention on the psychological harm which can result, applies to the many and varied forms which bullying can take, and takes into account the intent of the bully. In this way managers can be clear about where their responsibilities lie when dealing with a situation in which bullying is suspected.

We found Randall's definition most useful in this respect, because of its focus on the effects on the victim and the intentions of the perpetrator without using limiting words such as 'persistent':

> *Bullying is aggressive behaviour arising from the deliberate intent to cause physical or psychological distress to others.* (Randall, 1997)

Recognising bullying behaviour

Adams (MSF, 1994) stated that the power of the bully lies in making people remain silent through fear and, without prescriptive legislation, it is usually immensely effective. She pointed out that complaints often sound trivial when taken out of their original context, but it must be remembered that a constant barrage of criticism destroys self-esteem. It is only just beginning to be recognised as a cause of psychiatric injury.

According to Adams (MSF, 1994) typical bullying behaviour can include:

- Hovering over people like birds of prey pouncing, to torment their victim over trivia
- Constantly over-monitoring people's efforts
- Constantly undervaluing effort
- Persistent criticism
- Irrationally explosive outbursts
- Belittling people with personal remarks
- Spreading malicious rumours
- Withholding information
- Taking credit for other people's ideas
- Ignoring or excluding an individual by talking only to a third party to isolate another
- Setting objectives with impossible deadlines, unachievable tasks in the time given
- Removing areas of responsibility and giving people menial or trivial tasks to do instead
- Humiliating people in front of others.

Andrea Adams' work is amongst some of the earliest on this issue in Britain but the behaviours which she identifies have been reported frequently in almost every study on bullying behaviour.

> *You can kill a person only once, but when you humiliate him, you kill him many times over.* The Talmud

The RCM study (RCM, 1996) found the commonest forms of bullying behaviour to be intimidation, undervaluing of skills and humiliation.

Other forms included belittling of work, undervaluing effort, questioning of professional competence, excessive criticism, threats, blocking development/promotion, withholding information, overruling decisions, moving goal posts, refusing reasonable requests, ostracisation, malicious lies and abuse. These are typically female bullying techniques which are discussed in greater detail in Chapter 3.

Research into bullying has long been hampered by such lengthy lists of possible bullying behaviours. Hopefully, as research is consolidated and becomes more refined, this will become easier. To simplify matters, Rayner and Hoel (1997) categorise bullying behaviours into five areas:

- Threat to professional status
- Threat to personal standing
- Isolation
- Overwork
- Destabilisation.

Using the behaviours described in the RCM study, we will now see how they might fit into Rayner and Hoels' categories:

Threat to professional status

Can include belittling of work, undervaluing effort, questioning of professional competence and excessive criticism.

Threat to personal standing

Can include intimidation, humiliation, threats, malicious lies and abuse.

Isolation

Can include blocking development and/or promotion, withholding information and ostracisation.

Overwork

It is interesting to note that in the RCM study this was not reported as a form of bullying, but it can include such behaviours as undue pressure to produce work, impossible deadlines and unnecessary disruptions. It may be the case that midwives consider such pressures a 'normal' aspect of their work yet, as we will discuss later in this book, they are no less damaging to one's health. However, a failure to recognise a maternity department as a high-risk environment (and the staff within it as a high risk group), and a failure to have taken steps to implement effective strategies to reduce stress among the staff, could certainly be considered employer neglect, if not actual bullying.

Destabilisation

This can include undervaluing of skills, overruling decisions, changing goal posts, and refusing reasonable requests.

Comparison between studies is difficult, not least because of the problem of definition, which should become easier if the above categories are replicated in other studies. However, it is worth comparing the RCM study with the work by Quine (1999) because of an interesting anomaly in the category of overwork. The point about overwork is interesting. It would be too easy too assume that midwives never complain about being overworked but, as midwives, the authors are well aware that they do, and frequently! Overwork is definitely an issue for midwives, but perhaps they don't consider it a manifestation of bullying behaviour.

It must be remembered that this could also be accounted for by a difference in questionnaire design, but in Quine's study of bullying within a NHS Community Trust the most frequently reported bullying behaviours were:

- shifting the goal posts
- withholding necessary information
- undue pressure to produce work, and
- freezing out, excluding or ignoring.

In fact Quine states that if these four behaviours were taken in isolation the incidence of bullying in her study would still have been 32%.

Gender difference

Whilst Quine's study divides people up into professional groups, it is a pity that the study is not gender specific because there are interesting differences between male and female bullying styles. The chosen style usually results in the most harm to the victim, which puts a particularly nasty twist on the whole issue. For example the female bullying style hurts women more than the male style would, and vice versa. This proves that the intent is definitely to cause as much harm to the intended victim as possible.

Randall (1997) found that there were gender differences in bullying style, with women using 'relational' bullying more often. This will be explained more in chapter 3 but briefly, he suggests that because women are particularly dependent on having good relationships with co-workers and colleagues, the easiest way to hurt them is to threaten those relationships and exclude the victim from them. Female bullies, therefore, would tend to adopt techniques such as social exclusion.

Managers must bear in mind gender difference when handling complaints in this area. What women may consider bullying, men may not, and vice versa. This does not mean that the victim has not been psychologically harmed but it could affect the victim's perception of being taken seriously by the manager where the manager is a different gender to the complainant. There is the potential for this to be a particular problem in the Health Service where the workforce is predominantly female yet senior management is still predominantly male. For example, Randall points out that men and women view sexual harassment differently (see Chapter 3 – attribution theory) but states that because of the distribution of men in senior management the male view will predominate. This is thought to be a major factor explaining why women fail to use personal harassment procedures to address sexual harassment grievances.

At the moment society is divided between those who abhor workplace bullying and those who secretly admire or condone such behaviour. This is illustrated in comments such as:

temperamental behaviour often accompanies genius.

In a television documentary following the career of chef Gordon Ramsay (*Ramsay's Boiling Point*, Channel 4, from February 25th to March 25 1999), the subject is described alternately as:

a genius

and

a first-rate chef but a second-rate human being.

The Times described him as 'the new enfant terrible of the kitchen' (*The Times*, Sat February 20, 1999), a phrase couched in endearing terms. This bully's behaviour is inexcusable, though there are plenty of people who do make excuses for him. A member of staff who was sacked by him (apparently sackings happen at least once a night) defended him, saying 'he really was a very good chef'. The implication was that he couldn't be a very good chef without his violent outbursts, yet this is patently untrue because there are many great chefs who are even-tempered.

There is an analogy here with society's attitudes towards racism and sexual harassment. Those who were opposed to changing the legislation initially resisted all attempts to outlaw such behaviour and coined the term 'political correctness' in an attempt to trivialise the issues, discredit political opponents, and avoid having to change workplace attitudes and behaviour. Many people remember the character Alf Garnett in the television comedy *Til Death us do Part* whose behaviour is considered shocking and offensive by today's standards, but the reason the show was so popular at the time was that most people knew somebody exactly like him, who held similar beliefs and opinions about women, black people, Irish people and 'scousers'. Some still do.

If offensive behaviour is to be outlawed then bullies like Gordon Ramsay must realise that their behaviour is unacceptable. For this to happen people must stop defending such behaviour, genius or not, and Ramsay's peers and wider society must express genuine disapproval of such behaviour. One member of staff in Ramsay's kitchen was unfortunate enough to make a simple mistake and was immediately subjected to an explosive, violent, outburst of verbal abuse that would have made Alf Garnett blush. Under this barrage of abuse the individual concerned was more likely than ever to make a mistake. No one should ever think that they have to endure such abuse either in the pursuit of a career or in doing a regular everyday job.

The psychological effects of bullying can be devastating. It damages confidence in one's self and destroys careers. Victims lose self-esteem, confidence and faith in their ability to do anything. They may suffer anxiety and panic attacks. There is now legal recognition that psychiatric injury can result from the actions of another and that this is a form of actual bodily harm. This topic will be explored further in Chapter 5.

Bullying can lead to sleeplessness and various stress-related conditions such as post-traumatic stress syndrome, anxiety, migraine, skin disorders, back pains, stomach problems, and an increase in heavy smoking and/or heavy drinking. Some general practitioners have started to include workplace bullying on sick notes as a valid cause of ill health.

MSF (who incidentally represent many NHS staff) stated in their report:

> *Where management adopted a bullying approach the following consequences were likely:*
> – *Absenteeism due to stress*
> – *High staff turnover*
> – *Under-performance.* (MSF, 1994)

With absenteeism, desire to leave, increased job-induced stress, depression and anxiety rife throughout the NHS (MSF, 1994; RCM, 1996; Quine, 1999) it is imperative that, if the recruitment problems and sickness/absence within the NHS are to be permanently addressed, then the bullying culture that permeates the NHS must be addressed as a matter of urgency.

Victims can feel as though they 'ought to be coping' and that it is their own incompetence which is 'the problem'. An organisational culture can exist where 'problems' are ignored, because to acknowledge them may be interpreted as an admission of incompetence, and used by the bully as further 'ammunition' in his or her vitriolic attacks. Departmental or organisational goals can be sidelined as staff become engaged in 'defensive' activities to placate the bully and avoid provoking an outburst.

It is interesting to note that the MSF study found that, despite workplace bullying, high staff turnover decreases during a recession. This could mean that during times of recession when staff are unable to move on or change employment they are forced to suffer in a bullying situation for longer. The deleterious effects on health would be aggravated in such cases.

Where staff are ambitious or, for whatever reason, are highly motivated to succeed, they will neither challenge a bully who is their senior nor consider changing job or career.

Another television documentary, *Bullying Bosses* (ITV, September 1, 1998) featured chef Gordon Ramsay again, but this time the programme makers were expressing disapproval of his bullying tactics rather than glorifying them. Interestingly, the programme clearly demonstrated how much of his abuse student chefs were prepared to suffer because of their determination to succeed. The abuse and degradation which these particular student chefs put up with was also shocking:

F— off. Close the f——— door and clean the stairs.

During the documentary we referred to earlier, which was screened after this one, Ramsay can be seen watching the above documentary and laughing at his own behaviour. His family and colleagues were laughing too, which served to condone this behaviour.

It is hard to imagine that bullying is acceptable in any working environment, yet every day such behaviour goes unchallenged in many organisations including restaurants, hospitals, and the services. In recent years cases have been reported in the Army, Police and Fire Service. Typical bullying behaviour, as described above, is commonplace and the victim usually (though not always) holds lower rank within the organisation than the bully.

We discovered that, within the midwifery profession, the perpetrator may bully peers, junior staff, students and even women in their care. Bullying is particularly despicable, and is at its most psychologically damaging, when the tormentor has formal power which is subsequently abused. This is the case when midwives bully women for whom they ought to be caring, and when the statutory Supervisor of Midwives abuses this position to run a campaign of career and character destruction against a midwife.

At a conference on midwifery supervision Breda Seaman (1995) related her experience of what she termed 'poor supervision'. What she described as 'negative' midwifery supervision coupled with 'harassment and victimisation' was a first hand account of a long-term bullying campaign, executed by the statutory Supervisor of Midwives. Unfortunately hers is not an isolated case. During our research for this book we heard similar stories where Supervisors of Midwives had abused their position in this manner.

For the benefit of non-midwifery readers, part of the statutory Supervisor of Midwives' role is to ensure professional competence. Since there is no regulatory provision, the position is ideal for a bully who can use the supervisory role freely as an excuse to apply some of the bullying behaviours we outlined earlier, such as over-monitoring of people's work, questioning professional competence, blocking promotion, removing areas of responsibility and giving people menial or trivial tasks to do instead.

The Supervisor of Midwives has a statutory power to impose certain measures in cases of professional incompetence and, in the cases of the bullying supervisors reported to us, these 'measures' were actually bullying techniques thinly disguised under the name of 'supervised practice'. Unfortunately there is no requirement for a Supervisor of Midwives to prove a case for an individual midwife's incompetence before she or he imposes these sanctions.

Case study

Alison was a Staff Midwife working on the labour ward. She says she was bullied by a Community Midwife (Sister Jones) who was also her Supervisor of Midwives. Alison describes herself as having an 'easygoing bubbly personality' and feels that the 'cause' of the bullying was jealousy. She points out that she never prompted such behaviour and was never unpleasant to Sister Jones in any way.

Alison first discovered that Sister Jones was speaking of her in derogatory terms when a couple enquired whether Alison could deliver their second baby, as she had delivered their first. This couple were unimpressed when Sister Jones replied:

Oh you mean Mrs Stupid.

The next time this couple saw Alison they told her what Sister Jones had said.

Following this initial incident Sister Jones began repeatedly to tell Alison she was stupid, often in front of colleagues. She would read Alison's written records (on labour ward) and be over-critical in a sarcastic manner. Alison states:

She would try to put me down in front of colleagues and ignore my views in any discussions.

Alison feels that Sister Jones was using her professional power to criticise and manipulate her to the point where she felt 'powerless' to defend herself. Alison describes the effect as follows:

I began to lose confidence and my self-esteem reached an all time low, I was tearful, I could not make decisions at work, I basically felt unable to function, in the end I visited my local Samaritan group for counselling.

Alison informed her manager and also found support from another senior midwife. Following this she discovered that Sister Jones had bullied other colleagues.

Alison says the bullying, which continued for some months, has now stopped because she has moved to another area and doesn't see Sister Jones anymore. She describes Sister Jones as 'generally an aggressive person in nature and this is displayed when she communicates'. She continues:

Midwives in general do have a problem with 'power'. It is almost like a game of 'oneupmanship', and it is a constant battle. It makes you want to ask yourself what are these midwives like with the women and families they care for?

As Adams points out, setting people up to appear incompetent is a common bullying tactic. It must therefore be especially tempting for a bully who is in the position of assessing and monitoring professional competence, such as a Supervisor of Midwives or a line manager.

> *setting them [staff] up to look professionally incompetent is often the bully's way of getting rid of what he or she sees as the competition.* (Adams, 1992)

The traumatising effects of bullying are magnified when the person responsible for offering support and advice (the Supervisor of Midwives) colludes with, or is the bully. People in this situation are especially disempowered. They often lose all hope, feeling that they have nowhere else to turn. Additionally, most grievance procedures require the aggrieved party to pursue complaints through the managerial line. This can render the victim totally powerless and increase the power of the bully, in situations where the bully is the victim's line manager. In this situation the victim can live in constant fear of losing their livelihood, as the bully possesses the power to invent charges to bring disciplinary action against the victim. Abuse of disciplinary procedure was a common bullying tactic reported to us.

Some midwives told us that a bullying approach was 'deliberately' and 'systematically' adopted by Supervisors of Midwives and Midwifery Managers together, as a joint strategy to 'force' them to leave. Making an employee so uncomfortable that they are forced to leave is known legally as constructive dismissal, which will be discussed later in this book. However during the mid-1990s, when many NHS Trusts were trying to reduce their staff salaries bill, it was very convenient for a manager to be able to replace a 'G' grade midwife with an 'F' grade or lower. All the more convenient if the 'G' grade midwife left her employment early.

It was also reported to us that in some units, 'G' grade midwives were singled out. Their work would be scrutinised and over-criticised. Many would be accused of professional incompetence and their practice 'supervised' in the manner referred to earlier. In one example the midwife was informed that her practice was to be supervised by a midwife who had already been bullying her. The manager was aware of this and, indeed, colluded with the bully. When the midwife requested an alternative Supervisor of Midwives, her request was refused. In this particular case the Midwifery Manager and the Supervisor of Midwives together contrived to make life as difficult as possible for this midwife who was eventually forced to leave.

We received one rather disturbing report from a concerned Midwifery Manager (in a different region from the midwife mentioned above) who claims this topic was discussed at a regional meeting of Midwifery Managers in 1995. She says it was her understanding from the meeting that the number of 'G' grade posts was to be reduced by fair means or foul. She felt that there was an implication that constructive dismissal would be condoned, if not encouraged, provided it produced the desired results. This suggests that workplace bullying may have been widely adopted as a form of constructive dismissal during the mid-1990s.

Bullying is often adopted as a 'gagging' technique. In a department where staff are often bullied, or fear being bullied, genuine concerns about staffing levels and/or patient care can be effectively trivialised and sneered at.

It has been argued (Hadikin, 1998) that NHS Trusts were relying on the exploitation of midwives to introduce the recommendations of the Expert Maternity Group, *Changing Childbirth* (Department of Health, 1993). With no funding available for on-call allowance, special duty payments and/or excess hours payments (overtime), midwives were increasingly being pressurised into working long hours with endless nights on call, and without taking necessary breaks. Under such circumstances midwives risk making mistakes through tiredness, a situation that doctors acknowledged was dangerous when junior doctors' working hours were reduced, yet midwives are expected to press on and those who raise objections are often subjected to bullying.

> *Changing Childbirth was the political lever which trusts needed to 'shake up' a maternity department: increase staff flexibility, get rid of any 'dead wood' and, most importantly (for them), reduce the staff wages bill, whilst staying this side of the law and avoiding charges of unfair or constructive dismissal by issuing new employment contracts.* (Hadikin, 1997)

One midwife had cause to provide her manager with a formal notice of 'unsafe conditions for practice', as recommended by the nurses and midwives professional body the United Kingdom Central Council for Nursing, Midwifery and Health Visiting (UKCC). She was told by the Midwifery Manager that it was 'rude and unprofessional' to do so. This not only goes against management 'best practice' but breaks the Nurses and Midwives' Code of Professional Conduct (UKCC, 1992).

One of the authors witnessed an incident in which an experienced, highly respected, midwife returned from a meeting with her line manager in tears, purely as a result of how she was treated and spoken to.

> *I feel so stupid, it's like being a little kid again.*

Another midwife told us that she actually went as far as seeing the manager (who had been bullying her) to request that she be downgraded, in the hope that this would 'take the heat off'. It didn't. She went off on long term sick leave and eventually took early retirement.

Bullying behaviour is not reserved for individuals. When left unchallenged, some bullies become so arrogant they progress to bullying whole groups of staff together, even in front of witnesses. The longer that the bully remains unchallenged, the more they consider that they are right and believe they are supported by the organisational culture or by their immediate managers. The behaviour becomes 'custom and practice' and changing it becomes more and more difficult for the organisation, the victim and the bully herself.

Racial and sexual harassment will be mentioned in later chapters as they bring their own particular problems and have their own legislation. Both these aspects, though, also compound the effects of bullying.

In our study few midwives actually used the term bullying. They preferred words such as harassment, victimisation, being picked on, singled out, or intimidated. After hearing midwives' accounts of their experiences, and reading the MSF conference report (1994), it was clear to us that these midwives were being bullied. In the past, midwives who experienced bullying behaviour had no label to help them make sense of their experiences.

We hope that a clearer understanding of what bullying is and the impact it has on individuals and organisations, in conjunction with effective employment legislation to protect individuals, heralds the beginning of the end for the workplace bully. In the next chapter we look briefly at the history of the NHS, with a view to understanding how some of these bullying behaviours originated, before proceeding to look at the cultural factors which help perpetuate them.

Chapter 2

Historical and social factors
How the NHS bullying culture developed

*They had to be taught
to be good mothers.
Some of them were very
foolish and irresponsible.*

Leap and Hunter, 1993

Most of us will at one time or another have heard stories of Hospital Matrons and Ward Sisters who used to rule their domain with a rod of iron, terrorising staff and patients alike. Leap and Hunter (1993) interviewed women who worked as midwives during the early decades of this century and had this to say of the women they met:

We were often shocked... by the authoritarian manner of the midwives. Many implied that they would go into women's homes and lay the law down in order to 'educate' people.

Mollie T., a retired midwife tutor of that era (cited by Leap & Hunter, 1993), described her amazement that midwives continued to do so much and so well in adverse circumstances. In this context qualities such as bossiness and strictness were seen as being not only desirable, but necessary, to ensure midwives were 'tough enough' to do a difficult job. She also suggests that 'unfeeling' and 'bossy' women were attracted to midwifery because it offered independence. The attitudes and approach of midwives during this era must be considered in historical context. The midwives of the 1920s and 1930s were at the forefront of social reform.

Towards the latter end of the 19th century, and the beginning of the 20th century, healthcare was only one aspect of the wider movement towards social reform, which encompassed issues such as housing and sanitation. This era gave rise to strong characters such as Florence Nightingale, the Rathbones (who started the Public Health nurses to improve hygiene) and 'Kitty' Wilkinson of the Wash-Houses. These were the forerunners of the stereotypical 'bossy and interfering' Health Visitors and District Nurses. Many of these early 'community' roles were combined, with midwifery forming part of the role.

According to Flinn (1977), towns and cities of this period were filthy, unhealthy places. Mortality rates were high from dysentery, cholera, and consumptive disease. The Public Health Act was passed in 1848 and by the latter half of the 19th century (and well into the beginning of the 20th century) the main concern of local authorities was still primarily to clean up the squalid, filthy conditions within industrial towns and cities.

Of major concern to the social reformists was the 'condition of the working classes'. One of the aims of the early public health movement was to teach the working classes the value of cleanliness and hence reduce the extremely high mortality rates. Midwives, by then educated women under the instruction and supervision of the local authorities, were employed to instil 'good', clean, habits into the ignorant masses.

It is important to note that, at this time in history, the 'ignorance' of the working classes was a major issue on the political agenda. This precluded working-class women from becoming qualified midwives as they would have been considered unfit, and prone to spread ignorance, disease and dirty habits. The working-class 'woman-you-sent-for' was rapidly being replaced by educated, qualified, 'professional' midwives: from 'respectable', aristocratic and middle-class, backgrounds.

The philosophy of Victorian paternalistic philanthropy prevailed: the midwife (having received an 'education') knew what was 'best'. Working-class women were expected to do as they were told:

They had to be taught to be good mothers. Some of them were very foolish and irresponsible. (Leap and Hunter, 1993)

Public health inspectors and midwives alike were all part of this general public health movement. Though their visits may not always have been welcomed, the fact that midwives were seen as being able to help somehow excused their behaviour. Working-class women had no 'right' to question authority. The emergence of 'science' as the doctrine which would 'save mankind' was also reaching its peak in popularity at the turn of the century, with the advancement in anaesthetics, surgery and the discovery of microbes.

Some of the authority granted to these midwives was as a direct result of the Victorians' love of, and faith in, science. Midwives were considered 'scientific' because they were trained by the medical profession. Within the context of the public health movement, midwives were viewed as 'agents' of science; sweeping filth and degradation aside and issuing forth an era of light, knowledge and (more importantly) 'good' hygiene!

During this professionalisation of midwifery, midwives were involved in a political struggle for the control of childbirth with their powerful rivals, the medical profession. In addition to their 'tough' image, midwives also publicly adopted a powerful political strategy (Nettleton, 1995) to gain professional status and recognition.

Prior to the Victorian era, women worked alongside men in agriculture. Dairy workers (circa 1700-1800) are a particularly good example. Far from the romantic notion of the 'merry milk-maid' the reality was that the women who worked in dairies were likely to be strong, muscular women, capable of carrying heavy milk churns and turning huge cheeses. The work was long, hard and laborious.

This held no implications for their femininity or gender before the Victorian moralists came along. It was the Victorians who first suggested the idea that women were a 'weaker' sex and unsuited to certain types of work. This notion did not, however, appear to filter down to the lower classes of women, who were still expected to 'man' the workhouses and coal mines.

Class difference

Few working-class women managed to gain the necessary qualifications, but those that did weren't so unsympathetic to the working-class mothers in their care:

> *On the whole, the working-class midwives we interviewed appeared to have more empathy with the women they attended.*
> (Leap & Hunter, 1993)

Hunt and Symonds (1995) studied contemporary midwives at work in a modern maternity unit. Their work reflects women's expectations of midwives today. In their study some women found the terms used by midwives patronising but did not challenge this, as this was how they had expected midwives to talk. It appears that intimidating behaviour may have been present from the inception of the midwifery profession but has only recently been redefined as 'a problem'.

Sociological factors

Sociologists describe the process through which people learn the culture (values, beliefs, customs, rules and regulations) of their society as socialisation (Haralambos, 1987). In smaller groups, such as the professions, subcultures exist through which members identify one another and which differentiate members from the mainstream culture.

Leap and Hunter's (1993) description of the 'trials' which newcomers to the profession were put through, suggests that students learned intimidating behaviour as part of their socialisation into midwifery:

> *... we had a nurse there and she was rather strict and she said, 'if you don't take this castor oil, I shall hold your nose and pour it down your throat...'* (Leap and Hunter, 1993)

Blane (1986) suggests that senior members of a profession mould the new generation in their image, and that such a prolonged process of selection and socialisation makes professions stable and very conservative institutions. Professional traditions and customs would therefore be very slow to respond to social changes.

It takes approximately 30 years for traditions and customs to become established as part of any professional culture. This is because of the overlap of generations. Midwives who trained in the 1930s were still teaching students in the 1960s, and midwives who trained in the 1960s are still training midwives in the 1990s, hence technologies and skills may alter but ideas and culture can be up to 30 years behind! Especially since students may have new ideas but they have no influence on practice. Individual ethics and standards may differ but this 30 year cycle is one reason why it is so difficult to alter corporate culture. It may take a 20-year-old student the whole 40 years of her working life before her ideas and philosophies will imbue the corporate culture.

It appears that midwives both personally and professionally developed a strict, authoritarian image out of necessity, but that this became inextricably linked to their professional identity, as part of their professional subculture, and passed on to new generations in the form of tradition.

The harsh, ruthless, often cruel, attitude of early nurses and midwives was perpetuated through a training system which forced students to undergo a 'trial by fire' to test their resolve, character and discipline. The methods adopted to 'shape' newcomers to the profession was tantamount to bullying on a huge scale:

> *I found what every other nurse finds in those first few weeks – that scrubbing, cleaning, polishing, sluicing, bed-panning and*

who the hell do you think you are and what the devil are you doing here attitude from seniors are the basic laws on which ministering angels are created... if she never had an inferiority complex before, she will certainly develop one before the first week is over. (Leap and Hunter, 1993)

There are historical links between the Army and the nursing profession. Early nurses, including Florence Nightingale, worked within the context of Army field hospitals. When they transferred nursing principles, including the culture, to civilian hospitals they carried with them the attitude that 'nurse knows best'. The patients were there to do as they were told, if they expected to get better, whilst the students were there to be bullied, bellowed at and also (if they knew what was good for them) do as they were told. Consistent with the nursing profession's military history, patients and students alike were treated as newly-conscripted recruits, with qualified staff behaving like regimental sergeant-majors.

Nursing staff had no teaching skills and were expected to train students in the manner in which they had been trained themselves: by imposing strict regimes and discipline. The analogy with 'ministering angels' reflects early attitudes towards nursing: that is, with the emphasis being on 'self-sacrifice' and 'servitude'.

In addition to the traditional links with the Army, nursing had even earlier links with the Church and missionaries. Historically, caring for the sick, poor and crippled was the preserve of local parishes. The religious overtones can still be detected in the choice and use of language, as in the use of the terms 'ministering angels' and 'sister'. These imply that nurses and midwives are something more than human, which may explain why they were supposed to lead a convent-style lifestyle, denying themselves everything but the basics.

The Church was a historical recruiting ground for nurses and midwives, and was another institution where obedience, poverty and selflessness were paramount rules, especially for the Roman Catholic Sisters from a variety of callings. Missionary work, contemplation and prayer evolved into the caring professions with nuns (nursing 'sisters') requiring training and education in nursing, and for others in teaching and eventually social work. Their influence in continually putting others first and self last, with low pay and poor conditions, have permeated the NHS.

Other vocational professions were quick to shake off these influences but within nursing it suited the state-controlled NHS to continue to attract young and impressionable women and mould them into obedient servants of the state. The conditions placed on student nurses until the 1970s included being resident during training, wearing a uniform correctly and being punished for breaking minor regulations. Low pay and the reliance for lodgings, friends, entertainment and social support from within the profession kept nurses in their place and unable to challenge the system that controlled so many aspects of their lives. It was easier and more personally beneficial to 'play the game' according to the rules rather than upset the status quo.

When the supply of malleable young women began to dry up due to greater and more varied job opportunities, the authorities began to recruit a similar type of student who would not challenge the system because she was reliant on it, from the then commonwealth colonies and southern Ireland. Even in the 1990s we see recruitment from the Philippines to perpetuate a culture where nurses are expected to 'suffer' for their vocation. This can only continue an atmosphere of supporting tradition, not challenging injustices and becoming part of the nursing/midwifery culture. Those who do step out of line are soon brought to book, or leave.

Early nurses and midwives were expected to be hard, tough, unemotional individuals who could persevere under duress. Not being able to 'cope', being 'too emotional' or 'giving-in' to fatigue or ill health would all have been interpreted as signs of 'weakness of character' and one's suitability to the profession would have been questionable. This attitude is reflected in the following account by a retired midwifery tutor:

> *In the 1930s we lived in a small village on the Kent coast, and we had there what was called a Jubilee nurse... sent to... train as midwives... She had got terrible 'white leg' which must have been from childbirth followed by pelvic infection, and she used to get around the village on her own two feet, puffing and blowing and she must, at the time I remember, have had a heart condition, for she was always distinctly blue on exertion... She used to cover quite an area, at least two other villages along a seven-mile strip of the coast. She must have got there either by lifts or people coming to get her. She was in no state to cycle.* (Leap and Hunter, 1993)

Nurses and midwives had to be prepared to sacrifice their own time, health and even relationships (as nurses and midwives in those days were not allowed to marry or they were forced to leave the profession) for the sake of their 'vocation'. Indeed early claims for higher pay for nurses were instantly dismissed on the grounds that it would 'attract the wrong sort' to the profession. Thus working-class women were again disadvantaged: any woman who needed to earn a decent wage, could not do so in the nursing profession.

The 'jubilee' midwife in the above quote was evidently, by today's standards, unfit to practice, yet in her day she was respected and admired. Her cyanosis and breathlessness were signs of her sufferance and the fact that she continued to work in spite of her ill health was considered evidence of her dedication! The fact that this may have impeded her performance seems to have escaped the attention of her admirers. Such self-sacrifice, bordering on self-neglect, is not surprisingly reminiscent of martyrdom. This illustrates the moral context in which care was given during the Victorian period and such attitudes were still in existence until quite recently.

This quasi-religious atmosphere, where the deification and godlike status of doctors was coupled with the martyrdom of nursing staff, lent a good deal of authority to the nursing and midwifery professions who, in occupying the moral high ground and acting as 'agents' of God, deemed it appropriate to pass judgement. It must be remembered that during this era the Christian God of Victorian England was a God of 'hellfire and brimstone'. Such idioms as 'cleanliness is next to Godliness' and 'one must be cruel to be kind', were strongly held beliefs with their roots in fervent religious faith.

Once judgement was passed, mercy or punishment was expected. Gate-crashing working-class homes to rid them of filth was not considered rude: on the contrary, middle-class Victorians believed they were saving people's souls and in so doing were redeeming themselves by fulfilling their duty to the poor. Bullying patients and pupils alike appeared justified, as it was 'for their own good', and couldn't possibly be as bad as any punishment God would administer if their ungodly ways went unchecked. The popularity of science and the discovery of microbes fuelled this belief that right was on their side.

Moral concepts such as the 'deserving' versus the 'undeserving' poor can still be seen in healthcare today. Smokers, for example, are today sometimes refused treatment on the assertion that their condition is self-inflicted. Evidence of the sacrifice which nurses and midwives are still expected to make today can be seen in the fact that basic wages are relatively low and yet staff are still expected to work unpaid overtime with few or no meal breaks.

Aggression in mainstream culture

To place all this in context we must remember that the NHS is not alone in having to deal with conflict in the workplace. Overt acts of human aggression cannot be confined to the pages of a history book, since there is war and strife somewhere in the world almost every day. However, during peacetime, there have been periods in history when aggression has been socially acceptable and other periods, such as contemporary Britain, when it has been seen as socially unacceptable.

Ruthless, aggressive and cruel attitudes have been part of mainstream culture at various times and places throughout history, identifiable by their expression through mainstream politics. So much so that some psychologists have been led to question whether human aggression is, indeed, normal. This will be explored further in Chapter 3.

For example in the 1930s and 1940s, in Nazi Germany, Hitler held a fundamental belief in the 'survival of the fittest' (Rees, 1997). Rank and power were not earned but were 'taken' by overpowering any opponents. If a Nazi was ruthless enough to dispose of his opponents by any means, he was admired for it.

Hitler's attitude was mirrored in some of the management philosophies of the 1980s and early 1990s. Despite the presence of equal opportunity policies designed to encourage and facilitate the employment of disabled people, a ruthless attitude often prevailed:

> The current climate promotes such attitudes as 'if you can't stand the heat get out of the kitchen'. (RCM, 1996)

In many workplaces bullying managers are still often nicknamed 'Hitler'. The language people adopt often reveals their true feelings. Previously, managers who adopted such harsh attitudes towards their staff were not necessarily cruel or bad in themselves but were part of a generalised move in society which believed that you had to be pretty tough to do a tough job. Also the belief that so-called 'soft' people needed 'toughening up' was widely held.

Porteous (1997) claims burnout 'must not be confused with "cop-out"' which, he says, is:

> *finding excuses for poor performance... malingering, feeling bad, blaming external factors and acting the part of the perpetual victim to make life easy.* (Porteous, 1997)

This statement reflects the particular right-wing attitude which dominated certain aspects of British management culture. Whilst modern management philosophies, such as Human Resource Management, advocate genuinely open discourse with employees, there is still something inherently patronising about the way some British managers are interpreting the latest initiatives. There is a tendency to simply change a title, without examining the underlying values, systems and management practices.

> *... that peculiarly English genius for taking something American and subtracting from it its one worthwhile aspect, so that you end up with slow fast food* (Terry Pratchett)

Reluctance to relinquish control is evident in the way some staff development programmes resort to the covert use of organisational psychology, including psychometric testing and NLP (Neuro-Linguistic Programming). In a genuinely open, learning organisation there would be no need to resort to such measures, as organisational development would be 'owned' and available to all – the organisation as a whole would benefit.

A lack of openness and tolerance is often demonstrated by the overzealous application of sickness/absence policy. Whilst physical fitness is admirable, it is a philosophical step closer to Nazism to suggest that the sick or disabled should not be tolerated in the workplace.

Therefore, from a sociological viewpoint, aggressive and intimidating behaviour may be learned during socialisation into the mainstream culture or as one socialises into subcultures such as the midwifery profession or NHS management.

The origin of human aggression has been a question which psychologists have grappled with since the inception of psychology as a science. Relevant psychological research will be discussed in the next chapter but one theory which is appropriate here, in a sociological context, is that aggression can be a response to a hostile environment. The following paragraphs explore why women who work in a male-type hierarchy such as the NHS, despite the fact that female employees are the majority, may perceive their working environment as a hostile environment.

Power and authority

According to Nettleton (1995), the medical profession acts as a powerful agent of social control. It helps to enforce 'socially appropriate' behaviour by reinforcing values. The Protestant work ethic is an example. Doctors reinforce the concept of health as 'the ability to work' because of their role in 'validating' or giving permission to have time off work for illness. This conveys the message that work is preferable to idleness. The doctor's formal authority in this area is evidenced by the fact that in order to be excused from work, your release must be sanctioned by a doctor.

Nettleton describes the sexist ideologies which underpin the medical model of healthcare and suggests that the gendered nature of power, within doctor-patient interactions, can be a source of conflict. The doctor, for example, has a paternalistic role to play. Nettleton also notes the view that women employees within the medical system are just as likely to make unkind, sexist, comments as their male counterparts, since the medical model of care perpetuates gender stereotypes. This could equally apply to women working within such male-dominated hierarchies as the NHS, for example female doctors, nurses and midwives.

Where women resist medical control, Nettleton argues, they have experienced defensive, even hostile, responses. Taking these factors into account, both women workers and clients, ironically, could perceive a maternity hospital as a hostile environment.

Midwives recognise this hostility when clients resist medical control and request a home confinement or a natural birth without the 'benefits' of medical intervention. Sometimes the hostile attitudes of the medical staff are disproportionate to the request of the woman. In nursing, although to a lesser degree, it can be seen when patients refuse interventions such as chemotherapy, surgery or radiotherapy for terminal illnesses, preferring hospice care where aromatherapy and diet may be used to help relieve the symptoms. Relatives who request 'no resuscitation' for elderly relatives may unknowingly be challenging the medical man's belief in his own deity-like attributes and receive a discouraging response.

This swing in popularity back to the pre-scientific basis for medicine, using the older and sometimes forgotten remedies, relaxation, herbal preparations, and naturally prepared and grown foods, is a challenge to the professions that, whilst seen as a fringe activity today, is rapidly being subsumed into mainstream culture. This challenge is not just to the accepted medical practices but to the very control that a medical qualification bestows on those in charge of the health services. This control can be misused.

Male-dominated hierarchies

Before we go any further it may be useful if we examine the concept of male-dominated hierarchies and explore why this is considered relevant. Though we use the term 'male-dominated' hierarchies we mean the typical male 'style' of organisation which was originally devised and governed by the traditionally male institutions such as the Army, Church and government. Although organisations such as the NHS can be shown to have employed vast numbers of women, they did not typically occupy positions of power within the organisation and are not responsible for the design of the organisation's current management structure.

Hierarchical organisations such as the Army and the Church have a linear 'chain of command' and individuals working within the organisation each have a place on a 'scale' whereby they are 'superior' to those beneath them but 'inferior' to those above them. As mentioned earlier, hospitals inherited this management structure from the Army and, to a lesser degree, the Church. Rules such as 'disobeying a senior nurse is considered a disciplinary matter' kept everyone in their place whilst enforcing the formal authority of one's superiors.

This style of social and organisational structure benefits men whilst placing women at a disadvantage. When working within this male-type of organisational structure men are more likely to succeed and women less so. In organisations where this structure exists the top jobs, and hence the power and authority, are dominated by men despite the fact that women may represent the majority of the workforce. The powerful advantages which this structure affords to men can even overcome a situation whereby men are outnumbered by women to a vast degree. This is evident in the nursing profession in which, though the workforce is predominantly female, men proportionately outnumber women when it comes to senior managerial nursing and teaching posts.

Effects on women's communication

From both within and without, bureaucracies frustrate and oppress women's attempts at communication. A common example is where a woman decides to complain to her Community Midwife about aspects of her hospital care which upset or disappointed her. The Community Midwife might respond by saying:

if you want to make a formal complaint this is the procedure.

Procedure? This immediately frustrates the woman. She thought she was already expressing her view to someone (in a position of authority) who appeared to be listening and sympathetic, but she has just discovered the reality of bureaucracy: if she doesn't follow 'correct procedure' her opinion doesn't count. Midwives often feel the same frustration. On many occasions midwives approach their line manager saying something to the effect of 'some women don't seem to like this...' only to be cut short by the manager saying 'well, we haven't had any complaints'.

Women's views are invalidated unless women are prepared to follow male 'rules of engagement'. At best women see this as unnecessary 'red tape', at worst it is seen as a deliberate attempt to befuddle the issue, frustrate their attempts to improve the service and, worst of all, create conflict.

Female midwives working within the NHS, come up against the same barrier of 'procedure'. If a midwife is not happy with some aspect of her employment she is likely to talk to the most sympathetic supervisor or manager. But unless she follows 'grievance procedure' and formalises her 'complaint' her opinion is deemed not to exist. Women need a forum to voice their concerns and opinions, without having to feel that they are complaining, yet where they can expect their opinions and concerns to be taken seriously and acted upon. At the moment women are put into the position of complaining because they are told this is the 'Procedure-For-Being-Heard'. Many opt out and are deemed not to have a voice.

Linguist Deborah Tannen has spent many years studying not only gender differences in conversation but the impact this has on our society, culture and, more importantly, our dialogues in the workplace. It is for this latter reason that she is often invited to give keynote speeches on interpersonal skills at Human Resource Development conferences. In her latest book, *The Argument Culture*, she explains how the culture of conflict permeates western society and that conflict is often seen as the only route through which to address differences of opinion:

> ...*criticism, attack, or opposition are the predominant if not the only ways of responding to people or ideas.* (Tannen, 1998)

It is obvious that in a society which excluded women's input for hundreds of years, the established systems and structures are male-influenced. Without the ability to 'wipe the slate clean' and start again, the way forward is to retain the better aspects of the existing systems but to adjust them to be more suited to today's society.

Chapter 3

Why and how do bullies bully?

*A sharp tongue is the only edged tool
that grows keener with constant use.*

Washington Irving, *Rip Van Winkle*

Due to the impact and potential damage which workplace bullying can have within an organisation we have decided to devote this chapter to a discussion of the psychological factors which may have a bearing on this phenomenon. Managers at any level, where managing people is part of their role, will sooner or later have to deal with interpersonal conflict in workplace situations. As we shall see in this chapter, bullying does not necessarily have anything to do with conflict. There are factors which can predispose a person to become a bully and there may be factors in a victim's psychological make-up or body language which attract a bully.

We must emphasise at this point that by discussing such factors, in our attempt at understanding, we are in no way condoning bullying behaviour. Understanding a bully's psychological make-up does not detract from an employer's duty of care, and understanding that a victim may have psychological traits which bullies can pick up on does not imply that the victim was 'asking for it'.

Some psychological theories

It is interesting to note that in the RCM survey (1996) staff commented on 'aggression' from senior colleagues. Whilst we all have some idea of what aggressive behaviour is, why it occurs is a question which psychologists have grappled with for years. As we shall see, there are many theories on why human beings become aggressive. *The Concise Oxford Dictionary* (Allen, 1990) defines aggressive as both 'forceful' and 'self-assertive'. It is sometimes thought by senior managers that bullying is merely a problem of perception: the initiator feels that she is being assertive or being 'firm' but the recipient feels that it is aggressive. Is this possible, or is it an excuse on the part of a bully to try and deny that any intimidation was deliberate?

Carl Rogers (1989) points to the difficulty in establishing which exact behaviour variables lead us to perceive a person as 'cold', for example. Midwifery staff, observed in a study by Hunt and Symonds (1995), were said to have noted a 'warmer' atmosphere during the night shift. It is difficult to identify with any degree of precision just exactly what is being described when a person, or indeed an 'atmosphere', can be described as cold or warm. Yet these terms do hold a common meaning for all of us which we understand to mean a degree of friendliness, or approachability, and nothing whatsoever to do with temperature! So what specific behaviour variables lead us to form this impression?

Perception and Impression formation

Perception has been described (Clark and Keeble, 1995) as a complex process which not only involves the simple registration of light, sound and other sensory information but also incorporates the process of interpretation and attachment of meaning to the received information. The processing of sensory information is known as data-driven processing whilst the individual's interpretation of what is perceived and understood is known as concept-driven processing.

Factors affecting perception

The most obvious flaws in perception are those affecting the data-driven processes, such as a malfunction or reduced function in any of the sensory areas. For example, blindness permanently affects the receipt of visual stimuli whereas extremes of light or darkness, or tiredness, can temporarily reduce the clarity of visual stimuli. Data driven processes can therefore be affected by internal (personal) and external (environmental) factors.

Concept-driven processes are related to cognitive functions such as thinking and memory, and can be influenced by a variety of factors including moods, hopes, fears, memories, past experience and cultural expectations.

One of the most significant illustrations of this in a bullying context would be a nurse who had been a victim of bullying in childhood. Functioning as a fully mature adult he or she may be coping well and leading a fulfilling life but could respond and react differently on an emotional level to an incident at work. If this person encounters a member of staff or a patient who is shouting or verbally aggressive, their past experience may lead them to feel intimidated, and promote a learned emotional response to the intimidation; they may then fear their oppressor and this would influence their subsequent behaviour. Colleagues who observe their response may deem that the victim has overreacted whilst having little or no understanding of their background. In this example, the response of the victim would be a post-traumatic stress response, but nevertheless it is still an emotional reaction that has been influenced by the victim's concept-driven processes. Post-traumatic stress is, by its very nature, a concept-driven process.

Case study

A very senior midwife, Margaret, had been running her own department for several years and was well liked and respected by the past and present management teams. When she suffered from a complete physical and emotional breakdown, that apparently came 'out of the blue', her colleagues could not understand why this had happened and neither could she. She had always been a 'coper' and extended fairness and kindness to her junior colleagues and her clients.

A recently-appointed member of the management team, with a reputation for meeting goals regardless of the human cost, seemed to see Margaret as a personal challenge and began by moving staff from her department and replacing them with several newly qualified and less experienced staff. Many of these were part-time and on several occasions the department needed to appoint bank nurses to cover gaps in staffing levels. These were used by the manager to illustrate Margaret's inability to manage her department, to undermine her at unit meetings and generally to make her life difficult. Margaret found that going to work began to be something she dreaded, instead of looking forward to the satisfaction she had previously felt. In a short space of time she had changed from an efficient and happy midwife to an inadequate and nervous woman who found decision-making difficult. Her colleagues wondered why she did not stand up to the manager and demand that she had sufficient experienced staff to run the department. They began to talk about her inadequacies behind her back as they felt that she had let them down as well as the clients. After Margaret had gone off on long-term sick leave she began to talk to a counsellor. Margaret could not understand the rapid change in herself from being in control to being a victim. During therapy she explored other times in her life when she had the same feelings of fear and inadequacy. One of the most vivid memories that she had not faced for many years was of a Girl Guide summer camp. Margaret was a patrol leader and took the role very seriously. A new guide captain, who may have seen Margaret's efficiency as a threat, began to belittle her and undermine her at every opportunity. By the end of the week Margaret had decided to leave the guides. This decision was brought about by her feeling that she had no weapons to fight back when an older and authoritative person began to bully her. She had regretted the decision to leave for many years after that, but had never explored her feelings or her actions. The same feelings of being undermined, belittled and not in control as a midwife brought about by the new manager simply resurrected the feelings and in effect brought about the same resulting behaviour. Margaret wanted to leave, and knew she would regret it. What she had not learned from childhood experiences was how to face up to bullying, but she is not alone in this.

Both the bully's and the victim's behaviour patterns are often set in childhood and their childhood and adult experiences, combined with their inability to find alternative ways to resolve conflict, leads to their behaviour being carried on throughout their adult lives. It is important to note that we are not blaming victims in any way, but rather illustrating the interactive nature of a victim-bully relationship. The bully is always to blame, because the decision to bully is theirs, but they choose their victims carefully and if they don't get the desired response they move on to another victim.

It is when a victim produces the 'desired' behaviour that a bully feels powerful and continues a prolonged bullying campaign. So, although the bullying is instigated and perpetrated by the bully, there is often a particular characteristic in the victim which the bully has been looking for. In other words, the bully is taking advantage of a particular attribute in the victim's psychological make-up.

In examining the common myth that bullies intend no harm, but that victims misunderstand their intentions, we feel we must make a brief point about perceptual illusions. If a bullying incident is not intentional on the part of the bully, and the victim erroneously perceives it as such (as bullies so often claim!), this would be an error of perception on the victim's part. We feel that we ought to explain why this is unlikely, if not impossible, so that victims can be confident in reporting bullies and bullies can finally stop repeating this lame excuse! The next short paragraph explains why bullying incidents cannot simply be written off as a perceptual error on the part of the victim.

Perceptual illusions

There are some well-known examples of perceptual error, whereby people consistently misperceive visual stimuli (Clark and Keeble, 1995). A famous example of this is the 'reversible goblet' (see Figure 1) where the picture is framed in such a way that you could see either two faces or a goblet depending on your perception. Such studies have tended to focus on a single stimulus, visual or auditory. In social interactions, however, people receive a great number of stimuli simultaneously.

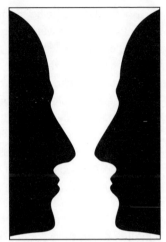

Figure 1

The more information we have from different sources, light, sound and touch, the less likelihood of our making a perceptual error. Perceptual errors occur most frequently with two-dimensional visual images presented in black and white. Dunbar (1996) discusses the importance of colour vision, for example, in primates and birds whose survival depends upon the ability to distinguish fruit from foliage. In social interactions we experience many varied stimuli from a variety of sources including sight, sound, smell, body language and many others. It is highly unlikely then, that perceptual error alone could explain feelings of intimidation within a complex interaction where one is receiving sensory information from many sources. It is therefore equally unlikely that a victim is mistaken in their belief that the bully intended to intimidate them. NHS managers would do well to remember this.

Impression formation

Following the above example one would form an impression of the other person. One may conclude that the person was angry, aggressive by nature or just childish. Whether positive or negative, the impression one forms would depend on one's overall perception and, once formed, impressions tend to stick. Hence the adage you only have one chance to make a first impression. We may not realise it but from our impressions and perceptions of others, we tend to assume motives for their behaviour.

Factors affecting impression formation

According to Clark and Keeble (1995) one of the problems with impression forming is that people make inferences from actions they have observed. Anger, they argue, is an inference from an observed facial expression. In other words, how do we know if someone is angry? We observe their expression and assume they are angry from the behaviour we observe. This is compounded if we already have a pre-formed impression of that person as a bad-tempered person. Clark and Keeble suggest that people have 'sets' of expectations, or principles, about other people which fill in the gaps in their knowledge and help to form a complete impression. These are known as implicit personality theories, an example of which is stereotyping. In our example then, our expectation that this person is angry is a result of our pre-formed impressions and the assumptions we make from their behaviour. Both of which can be wrong.

Stereotyping

Stereotyping is another means by which we may judge people inaccurately. Hicks (1995) conducted an interesting experiment with two groups of midwives who were to interview an imaginary candidate. The control group were given a description, comprised of six adjectives, including the term 'good clinician'. The experimental group were given the same description except that the word 'clinician' was replaced with 'researcher'. The groups were then asked to identify which character traits their candidate possessed. The experimental group thought their candidate would be more ambitious, a poorer communicator, less kind, stronger, more logical, less emotional, more confident, less popular, less compassionate, more rational, more organised, and more analytical than the candidate described as a good clinician!

Hicks' experiment shows how much we assume about a person based on a stereotypical image. It also demonstrates how one makes assumptions despite never having actually met the person, and how much can be assumed from just one small piece of information. The qualities 'less kind' and 'less compasionate' show that even aggressive characteristics such as ruthlessness were perceived to exist in an imaginary person.

Hicks had replicated an older experiment by Asch (1946). Following his original experiment Asch developed his cognitive organisation theory, in which he argues that people try to form consistent impressions of a person as a complete unit, despite sometimes meagre evidence. He used the term 'central traits' to describe qualities such as 'cold' which people used to form impressions. He showed that, to gain a consistent overall impression, people would try to avoid mixing positive and negative central traits. For example, people would find it hard to imagine that a 'good nurse' could also be a 'cruel' person.

Nurses and midwives are associated with the image of dedicated, caring, vocational people and because of this are often exploited into taking on extra work, shifts and responsibilities. The one who complains or refuses is thought to be a 'bad' nurse or midwife, who puts her own needs before the needs of the patient or the service. Somewhere these two needs have become interchangeable in people's minds and the nurse or midwife is made to feel guilty for wanting to be away from the workplace. Emotional and career blackmail is used to force individuals to fit into the corporate agenda. Threats of blocking career progression or study leave have been reported to us by all grades of staff, and for vulnerable people who need secure salaries these are very real threats that make people react in the way that the bully demands.

Today's society is becoming ever more image conscious and image influenced. We live in an era in which our minds are bombarded with visual imagery via magazines, television and the Internet at an unprecedented level. A whole new profession of image consultants has developed, with people advising on hair style, clothes, voice production, colours and make-up. These consultants work mainly with women although men also consult them when in the public eye, such as when the House of Commons is televised. People therefore acknowledge the power of image today in certain circumstances but should also be aware of the image they portray when at work.

The selected role must be backed up by image, otherwise mixed messages are being given to observers. For example, a nurse instructing a mother in asthma treatment for her child may consider that she is doing a good job getting the message across. But if she also smells of smoke due to a cigarette addiction the message is warped by the mixed image coming into the mother's consciousness. The efficient nurse who talks about her 'night-clubbing' the previous night may also be giving mixed images to the patient, and the interpretation may be different with different patients depending on the age, experience and expectations of the client.

These mixed messages of image versus expectations combined with dress, voice, words and body language can serve to confuse and also to undermine the power differential between people.

Here we briefly mention some theories which may sound familiar yet also have a part to play in perception formation:

self-fulfilling prophecy

people may expect certain behaviour and may act in such a way as to actually provoke the behaviour they expect.

projection

people assume that others will behave in the same way that they do and 'project' characteristics such as aggression onto them.

the halo effect

one's initial (positive or negative) impression influences future overall impressions.

actor-observer bias

one sees ones' own behaviour as a response to one's environment and circumstances but one attributes the behaviour of others to their disposition.

I'm in a bad mood because I'm having a bad day, you are just bad-tempered by nature!

Nowhere is this more evident than when looking at the friction which sometimes arises between full-time and part-time staff, or between staff with children versus staff without, who may have older dependent relatives who are just as demanding and a similar tie. The full-time staff are heard to complain 'She uses the children as an excuse not to work at weekends' (or holidays), but the working mother considers that she is doing a good job rearing her children and being part of the caring professions.

Some excuses are acceptable to one person who may have similar problems and not to another. For example, to say to a car driver that you were late for work because the bus was late may bring a sharp retort, but to say it to a similar public transport using member of staff may well attract sympathy and understanding. A person who has never suffered from migraine or period pains may be less sympathetic to a sufferer than someone who does.

Attribution theory

We will devote a little more space to this theory because, as will become evident, it is particularly relevant to bullying and harassment. Heider (1958) suggests that people do not merely observe others' behaviour but attribute a motive: why did he or she do that? He suggests that one's perception of why a person committed a certain act influences one's behaviour towards that person. Furthermore, it is only when one attributes a behaviour to an internal cause that one makes a judgement about the person's disposition. For example, if a midwife was late for duty because her car broke down, this is an external cause, but if she was late because she overslept, this is internal and one would make a judgement about her disposition from it.

Case study

Judy and Elaine had gone through basic training together and had become firm friends both in and out of work. When a vacancy for a G grade became vacant they both applied and Judy was appointed. Elaine went through the motions of congratulating her but really felt that she should have got the post. Shortly after this Elaine's marriage was in difficulty and she really missed Judy's support and friendship. At work Elaine began to make small errors and resented what she perceived as interference and criticism from Judy. Judy assumed that Elaine's behaviour was all down to jealousy about her appointment and that she was deliberately lowering her standards to put her, Judy, in a bad light. Their differences and suspicions soon overflowed so that the rest of the team began to take sides, though no one knew all the background, just the assumptions that each had made from observing behaviours. Judy found it impossible to manage the team and this was reflected in her increasing stress and attempts at control. Elaine felt victimised by Judy's behaviour and began to look at each incident as further evidence of her as a bully and herself as a victim. The outcome of this unhappy but far from rare tale is that Judy applied for a new post where she could manage a team of relative strangers whose assumptions were based on performance and not on vindictive gossip. Elaine found the stress of her divorce combined with the loss of her own self esteem forced her to leave the job she had previously loved and she became a part-time practice nurse.

Clark and Keeble (1995) describe a self-serving bias in self-attribution, whereby one attributes one's own 'good' behaviour to internal causes and one's 'bad' behaviour to external causes.

In addition to this, Shapiro (1981) notes a gender difference in self-attribution. He claims that women have different attributional styles to men, in that women would attribute personal success to unstable, external causes and personal failure to stable, internal causes. Shapiro links this with women's increased tendency to suffer from depression, because it is evidence of paradoxical logic. For example, if success is outside one's control, how can one be held responsible for failure?

Attribution and sexual harassment

Randall (1997) makes the important point that such gender differences in attribution, combined with the fact that men occupy senior management positions in greater numbers, often leads to the male view predominating on senior management boards.

The gender difference in attribution suggests that men are likely to believe the victim of sexual harassment was 'asking for it' or was provocative. The distribution of men on senior management teams means the male view will predominate. Also, where harassment policies are written in gender-neutral terms they fail to take account of the sexual differences in the interpretation of social/sexual harassing behaviour. This can militate against the most frequently harassed sex. Harassment procedures become under-used as women fail to take up grievances relating to sexual harassment because of the likelihood that senior management would relate more to the male view.

In deciding the motive behind people's actions and behaviour, one of the most common assumptions is in attributing an action to that person having a particular attitude.

Attitudes

Clark and Keeble (1995) suggest that there is a preoccupation within health education with people's attitudes to health because it is assumed such attitudes influence behaviour. However, they argue that there are inherent difficulties in establishing this relationship, namely that attitudes are internal and unobservable. Attempts to measure attitudes have centred on self-assessment which is not considered accurate unless it can be confirmed by observation. According to Clark and Keeble statements such as 'I don't like your attitude' assume that attitudes can be inferred from actions. They note that compliance with the behaviour norms of a membership group, such as midwifery colleagues, can lead to a shift in private attitudes. This supports Ingham and Fielding's (1985) observation that the strong pressures to conform to institutionalised norms are such that 'negative' behaviour prevails despite positive attitudes among individual staff. Personality, socialisation and group membership influence attitudes.

Peer pressure

Contemporary studies are beginning to acknowledge the importance of peer influence in human behaviour. Whilst the concept of peer pressure has always been acknowledged it had rather been marginalised, with early psychologists placing greater emphasis on the home and parental style as the major influences on personality and behaviour. However, according to Harris (1995), peer influence is possibly the most influential factor that makes us behave the way we do. Human beings are group animals, and we behave differently according to which group we are in and our own position within that group. The family is just one of the many groups to which we can belong. We will discuss more about group relationships and loyalty ties later, but it is important to note this shift in emphasis and to understand that now, in the light of our understanding of the importance of peer influence, bullying takes on a different aspect as possibly the main method of social control within human groups.

It is interesting to note how students or new staff behave in order to fit in with the culture of the organisation as they see it. The new member of staff observes the established organisational or professional culture, often without realising it. Attitudes of existing members to each other and to the medical and ancillary staff are observed, as are attitudes towards the clients. In an effort to 'fit in', and not to draw attention to oneself, it is easier and more desirable to become one of 'the gang'.

Nowhere is this more evident than in the armed forces or the police service. From basic training onwards, the main aim is to prevent free-thinkers from questioning orders and protocols, and to form a body of people who not only dress the same but think the same and act the same.

Fortunately nursing and midwifery is now moving away from this form of 'training', but pockets of it still exist. Many of us can remember moving from Staff Nurse/Midwife to Sister and promising not to become like 'one of them'. Within a short time however, the responsibilities of the role and the expectations of the organisation erode personal resolve and you become like 'them'. However in the mind of the individual no such changes have occurred and it is difficult and sometimes hurtful when others respond to the image rather than the person. Picking up on the attitudes and culture of an organisation is insidious and unless others point out changes the individual is often unaware of them. One of the authors was told at three Individual Performance Reviews that she was not ruthless enough to be a manager that suited the ethos of the organisation. It seems that image and portrayal can sometimes go against common decency and respect.

Case study

Paula, a Staff Midwife at the time, describes her experience in terms of 'lack of compassion', 'cold-heartedness' and 'thoughtlessness' rather than bullying or harassment. She describes commencing a post, as a newly-qualified Staff Midwife, at a hospital other than where she trained. The first six months went well and the midwives were friendly and supportive, but then her mother became terminally ill with cancer. Though her parents lived thirty miles away, the family relied on Paula to provide basic nursing care and liaise with Macmillan nurses; because she was the eldest daughter and because of her nursing background, it was felt she could understand technical jargon and explain it better to the family.

During this time she 'threw herself into her work' as a means of escape: she describes herself as 'working hard, getting involved in various projects and studying for a diploma'. She states that she informed her manager of her mother's illness but only to explain why she wasn't 'her normal self' - she did not request any time off.

Her mother died seven months after diagnosis. During the latter four months Paula was on labour ward. She states that she found it difficult 'not clinically, but emotionally', she found it 'hard to be pleased for new mothers and sharing in their happiness' and she expressed anxiety at being able to give women 'the standard of care I normally would'. She states:

It broke my heart and was emotionally exhausting.

During this period she mentioned her feelings to the senior midwife on labour ward and was told to 'pull herself together and be professional'. She felt this was exactly what she was doing. She asked for a transfer to either antenatal clinic or the antenatal ward, making arrangements to swap with another Staff Midwife, but this was refused. At this point Paula considered handing in her resignation and leaving. She states she couldn't talk to anyone, she felt like 'a leper', if she walked into a room the conversation would stop. She thinks people were 'probably anxious that if they asked me how I was I'd burst into tears'. She states:

In my naiveté I thought caring professionals could offer me some support but interpreted their response as apathy. I think now I recognise it as 'normal'.

She was also asked to go on night duty during this time. Normally she would have volunteered but felt at this time it was 'adding insult to injury'. She tried to negotiate a flexible arrangement, to enable her to continue to care for her mother, such as three nights on and three off but this was refused. She had to work eight nights on and seven off.

One night, when her father rang at 04.00 hrs, Paula feared the worst. He had never called work before. The Midwifery Sister who took the call said 'Your dad's on the phone, can you tell him personal calls should come through on the other number. You shouldn't have personal calls at work.' Her mother was in pain but already disorientated and her father had been afraid to give any more analgesia, and wanted her support and advice.

This particular Midwifery Sister had known the circumstances and the delivery suite was quiet that night. Paula asked if she could leave early and make the time up later. This was refused.

Her mother died later that week. The Midwifery Manager was inflexible, allowing only the minimum three days compassionate leave yet, because it was a bank holiday weekend, the funeral was delayed for almost a week. Paula informed the Ward Sister that she wouldn't be back on duty until after the funeral and that she'd take excess days as annual leave. The Sister said: 'OK, I'll let your colleagues know'.

Paula had thought there might be some expression of sympathy or compassion and couldn't understand why the staff were being 'so horrible' to her:

I certainly hadn't made a meal of having a dying mother... I had taken no sick time and only once (on nights) asked a favour to go early.

Paula describes 'the final insult' occurring on the day of her mother's funeral. The manager, who knew the funeral was that day, asked the Ward Sister to ring and ask when she would return to duty. Paula answered the telephone just as the hearse arrived. 'I'm afraid I swore and was less than pleasant', she recalls. On her return to work she was called to the Sister's office and reprimanded for her rudeness on the telephone.

Shortly after this time Paula left midwifery to take up another post and, as she writes:

was ecstatic not to have to work with these dreadful women again.

The above events happened around 1991. Since then, Paula has worked with people outside midwifery, and has recently returned as a midwifery lecturer. She states:

I can see a big difference between the way I respond to people, challenges and situations, compared to the way my midwifery colleagues do... often they seem less assertive, more cautious and terribly anxious at causing any offence. This seems to inhibit much of their creativity, natural warmth and dynamism... One iota of love, compassion and/or genuine concern would go a long way.

Paula does not claim that she was bullied, rather that the attitude of her colleagues (which she describes as lack of compassion, cold-heartedness, and thoughtlessness) during a bereavement increased her distress at a time when she would have expected support from them. It is interesting to note that she had expectations of support from this membership group which the group obviously did not feel obligated to. In contrast the group was overtly hostile, possibly to emphasise the point that they were not available to offer support.

In this example the midwife was newly-qualified but was working in a unit where she had not trained and hence she was a stranger to the staff. Her failure to adopt the dominant culture within that particular department was as a result of her being new and, having been preoccupied with her mother's illness, she may have failed to notice differences in the norms, values and beliefs. It is an excellent example of how nurses and midwives can use ostracisation and isolation as a powerful informal sanction.

Human aggression

Intimidating behaviour is often perceived as an expression of aggression. It may therefore be useful to examine some general theories on human aggression at this point.

Whether aggression is instinctive or learned is debatable and there is evidence to support both arguments. Storr (1970) claims that aggression is instinctive and, perhaps more importantly, inevitable under certain circumstances. Storr's arguments centre on the concept that aggression is necessary to enable us to compete and that the more competitive a situation is, the more aggressive we will become. In his view there is a direct relationship between aggression and competition. Other psychologists, such as Reich (1976) and Bandura (1977), maintain that aggression is learned. Bandura's social learning theory suggests that observation of behaviour in others and subsequent reinforcement is important in areas such as sex-role stereotyping. Therefore repeated images of macho male images portrayed through the media will ultimately lead to young boys becoming more aggressive. This is the theory behind the argument that watching increasingly violent videos and films will lead to a more violent society.

Storr's explanation of the motivation to compete is similar to Adler's mastery-drive theory (cited by Child, 1986) in that Adler suggests people are driven to succeed to avoid feelings of inferiority whilst Storr suggests that people are driven to compete by their basic insecurity. Inherent in both theories is the assumption that 'men' [sic] have an instinctive desire for control, mastery and superiority. However, Storr differs from Adler in one significant point. Adler believed that ultimately the needs of the group or society would supersede the needs of the individual. This implies that individuals have an element of control over their competitive urges and are capable of self-sacrifice.

In contrast, Storr argues that 'men' [sic] are motivated to form alliances only because of their basic vulnerability and insecurity, but that ultimately the needs of the individual will take precedent over group needs. Hence his conclusion that conflict and aggression are inevitable.

Psychologists working in the latter half of the 19th century and the early part of this century had little information on women and the information they had was coloured by their beliefs about the nature of women, namely that they were weaker and less aggressive than men. More recent work is just beginning to unravel the psychological differences between the genders. In terms of social interactions, Tannen (1995) points out how women tend to look for similarities and create networks of 'sameness' whereas men differentiate and create hierarchies based on superiority or inferiority. Given Tannen's insight into gender it is not surprising that Storr and Adler came up with the theories they did!

The Heresy factor

> *Conformity, based on close identification, at first promises reassurance, but easily becomes a restriction upon freedom to those who need to assert an individual point of view.* (Storr, 1970)

Storr argues that where people form alliances based upon strong ideologies, such as the early psychoanalysts Freud and Jung, security is only gained whilst all are in exact agreement. When an individual differs only slightly in their beliefs they are subjected to the most aggressive intolerance of all because they represent the greatest threat to the faith of the group as a whole. Storr claims that identification involves dependence which, in turn, leads to vulnerability to attack (from those upon whom we are dependent). Any divergence is a threat to inner security and produces aggression because it is interpreted as an attack. He believes that where associations are based on close identification, splitting is bound to occur and is inevitably accompanied by aggression. Heretics are therefore persecuted because they, more than anyone, threaten the security of the believer.

This has implications for managers during organisational change and managers of teams: if Storr's theories are applied to professional alliances then aggression between colleagues is inevitable, and the more competitive a situation is, the more aggressive. It's not so much a case of 'if' but 'when'. The greatest danger comes from colleagues who are almost, but not quite, in exact agreement. Given a situation which increases tension, such as an organisational change, and they can suddenly be having a major fight over what seems to everyone else in the team to be a relatively minor point.

Evidence of such competition in midwifery was described in 1936:

> *She got a job the following year, but she never forgave me in all the time we worked together for getting the first job! She was a real thorn in my side. The reorganisation caused a lot of friction.*
> (Mary W. cited by Leap and Hunter, 1993)

The implications of this for midwifery teams is that the cohesiveness of the team is likely to be threatened by the destructive effect of competition between individuals within the team.

Some recent theories on primate behaviour offer an interesting perspective on team psychology, peer influence and our reasons for forming collaborative relationships. Whilst it would be unwise to assume that information from animal studies can always be extrapolated to human situations, they often form the basis of behaviourist theories of psychology such as Pavlov's and Skinner's (cited by Child, 1986). Dunbar's (1996) theories on human social interaction deserve consideration here, because the social interactions of great apes and humans have important similarities, and research on the behaviour of great apes has not been limited by the same ethical considerations as research into human psychology.

Dunbar analyses and collates information from the biological, zoological and psychological fields to formulate his theories. He postulates that social interaction forms the basis of human societies and is the stimulus for the evolution of language. He observed collaborative behaviour in primates and claims that behaviour which benefits the group is necessary for survival and therefore takes precedent over any individual needs. He argues that human social interaction evolved as a mechanism to facilitate the collaboration required to survive increased predation as the early hominids ventured further out onto open plains away from the protection of the forest. At this point in evolutionary history, group survival was a priority over individual needs.

Collaborative behaviour: team psychology

Collaborative behaviour is still necessary for survival amongst the tribes inhabiting the Masai Mara in Africa. A Masai chief, interviewed by the one of the authors, explained how any one Masai warrior would be prepared to sacrifice his own life to protect the village from predators. Yet it is not only the village people he is protecting, it is the livestock, which are in many ways deemed more important! It is often the youngest warriors, who are still expected to 'prove' their worth, that are assigned this task of protecting the domestic cattle herds from wild predators. It is only after a confrontation with a predator, and if the warrior survives the encounter, that full status as a warrior, and the respect of other warriors, is earned. This is not only a rite of passage but is also an important way of instilling the concept that the individual's life is considered less important than the protection of the livestock which sustain the life of the whole community.

> *Young Masai warriors volunteer to throw away their spears and act as bait for a cornered lion. By walking in towards it holding his shield before him, the warrior forces the lion to jump him; his companions can then spear the lion in relative safety. By the time they have done this, however, the lion's hind claws – scrabbling for purchase beneath the young man's shield – have done their best to disembowel him. If he survives, he is feted as a hero of the village and becomes a much sought-after prize among the girls looking for husbands.* (Dunbar, 1996)

In pre-industrial agricultural or hunter-gatherer societies, communal needs took precedent over individual needs, as illustrated in the example above. It is difficult though to say without doubt that it is merely exposure to media imagery which increases violence in industrialised societies. There have also been political movements such as capitalism which encourage fierce competition and individualism. The effects of this have coincided with any effects from media imagery. Perhaps the key to understanding individual aggression lies in whether a particular individual perceives that they are 'included' or an 'outcast' from the larger society or group.

In contrast to Storr (1970), Dunbar's work supports Adler's view (cited by Child, 1986) that group needs will ultimately take precedent over individualism. Therefore competition among individuals within a team need not necessarily lead to potentially destructive, intimidating and aggressive behaviour. According to Dunbar the important factors are loyalty ties.

Teams, group ties and kinship

The team concept, as a collaborative structure for the organisation of midwifery care, has been proposed as the way for the future (Flint, 1993). This is the case in many organisations now, where the effective management of teams is deemed key to the achievement of corporate objectives. However, whether one is prepared to forego personal needs in deference to group needs could be dependent on the structure of the group, and one's perceived commitment and responsibility to other group members. Where midwives (or staff) are placed into teams not of their own choosing and/or against their wishes they may not have any loyalty or commitment to the group and, perhaps more importantly, to team objectives. Where midwives have been ostracised from the group, like Paula in our earlier case study, they may never regain any loyalty or commitment to the group and, as in our example, may need to move otherwise they could sabotage team initiatives.

Clark and Keeble (1995) distinguish between membership groups and reference groups. A membership group is where one is simply a member by nature of a particular characteristic or qualification, whereas reference groups are those where the values and standards are important to one.

Which category a team falls into depends upon the perception of an individual. For example, a midwifery team could merely be thought of as a membership group which one is a member of merely by virtue of one's work, yet it may become a reference group if the group standards and values become important to one. It is possible therefore that the approval of the team is more important to some members than others, and team members have differing levels of commitment to the team goals.

Time span is also important: people can make a team effort easily on a short project, but if forced to spend prolonged periods of time with people not of their own choosing the cracks begin to show. The analogy with prisoners is perhaps the most obvious here. Also, groups bound by family/kinship ties are stronger than other groups. This is evident in the research by Daley and Wilson (1988) who demonstrated that people are 20 times more likely to murder an unrelated person living with them than a genetic relative – bad news for lodgers!

According to Dunbar (1996) the network of ties and loyalties within a social group is more important than was previously thought. He suggests the primary reason for forming social groups is to reduce the vulnerability of isolation by developing a collaborative network of reliable support upon which one can call when threatened. Choosing the members of this group and ensuring their reliability is of prime importance.

Whilst it has been well documented that people can work effectively in teams (Adair, 1987; Oakland, 1993; Flint, 1993) the relative importance of the interpersonal relationships within teams has probably been undervalued. Emphasis has often been placed on the roles people play within teams (Oakland, 1993; Flint, 1993) at the expense of the ties and loyalties between team members. The relationships within teams, the ability to choose and the importance of feeling secure and supported within a team have been seriously underrated.

The power profile

Dictatorial bosses can be hell to work for: But, unfortunately for you, they are often the movers and shakers of the business world. So it may be more instructive to learn how to deal with one, than to moan or resign in disgust. (*She* magazine, September 1995)

When one considers some of the professions which are most often associated with workplace bullying, such as the army, police, fire service, catering/restaurants, managing directors, doctors, nurses and midwives, it is hard not to make an association between bullying and power. As with most debates on human behaviour, we often ask ourselves if people were born like that or have they learned to become a bully. This 'nature versus nurture' debate has continued among psychologists and sociologists for years and it is most likely that the answer lies in a combination of the two.

We mentioned earlier how people's behaviour is affected by their peers and the culture within which they work and live. This next section discusses the work of some of the psychologists who have studied whether such characteristics are intrinsic elements of the personality from birth. Much of this research was dismissed at the time due to errors in the structure or design of the research but, many years later, these theories are currently enjoying a comeback as we discover that environment cannot explain all human personality characteristics. Many of these early studies are being replicated by contemporary psychologists with a better knowledge of research design.

Explicit personality theories

It has been suggested (Eysenck, 1965; Kline, 1981) that there are dimensions of personality, each with a predisposition towards certain behaviours, for example extroversion, neuroticism and psychoticism. Eysenck describes each dimension as a continuum: extroversion/ introversion, neuroticism/stability, and psychoticism/normality. The psychotic dimension is particularly interesting when discussing the topic of workplace bullying.

Kline (1981) suggests that a person who scores high on the psychotic scale will be solitary, uncaring of people, troublesome, lacking in human feeling and empathy, thick-skinned, insensitive, cruel, inhumane, hostile and aggressive. After the Allitt enquiry (Department of Health, 1994) it is easy to see how disgraced nurse Beverly Allitt obviously displayed psychotic personality traits, but it is often easier to view these situations with the benefit of hindsight. Hopefully this chapter will offer some insight for managers into the types of people they may be required to manage.

There have been various attempts to categorise personality into 'types'. According to Shapiro (1981) 'lack of conscience' and 'cruelty' can be characteristics of a sociopathic or psychopathic personality, whilst aggression is typical in the 'Type A' personality.

Adorno et al (1950) compared prejudiced people with non-prejudiced people and concluded that there was an authoritarian personality, the characteristics of which were: to be narrow-minded, rigid, submissive to authority, sexually inhibited, intolerant of ambiguity and politically conservative.

In considering the application of these theories to healthcare management, the possibility that any of the psychotic personality types could account for the behaviour of a nurse or midwife is almost impossible to imagine. This is because, as we mentioned earlier, we find it hard to reconcile two such opposing character traits in one individual: because nurses by definition are supposedly caring, we cannot imagine they may be cruel psychopaths. Yet, again with hindsight, Beverly Allitt's managers must have wished that they had considered this possibility. The recommendations of the Allitt enquiry are outlined in Chapter 6.

The bully

Bullies are always aggressive individuals who intend to cause pain or the fear of pain. (Randall, 1997)

Other than those mentioned above, there is no formal personality classification of 'A Bully'. Rather, bullying behaviour is likely to be one aspect of a more complex psychopathic or authoritarian personality. As experts disagree over whether all bullying is intentional or not, this leads us again to question what exactly is bullying? For the purposes of this book we have adopted Randall's definition as one which is probably the most useful as a working definition to assist managers to assess their priorities when faced with a bullying situation among their staff (see Chapter 1).

Randall is of the opinion that intent is the key factor in bullying: that aggressive behaviour does not have to be regular or repeated for it to be bullying behaviour, provided that the behaviour was intended to cause harm or fear. Randall points out that bullies must have an expectancy that their behaviour will cause such fear or harm, otherwise they wouldn't do it! Randall distinguishes between 'affective' aggression, which is aggressive behaviour where strong emotions are involved, such as an outburst of rage; and 'instrumental' aggression, which is where no emotion is involved and the aggression is cold and calculated, like psychopathic behaviour.

Randall has spent many years studying bullying in children and has possibly done more research on this topic than any other psychologist. He is a leader in the field of bullying research. Possibly the most important conclusion which he has reached to date is that bullying children become bullying adults, and are likely to be wife and child batterers.

According to Randall, bullies are made, not born. He describes a bullying personality as one which fails to develop normally in childhood. Aggression is common to all young children, yet the majority learn how to convert this aggression into assertiveness by the development of social skills which combine assertiveness with the inhibition of aggression.

The victim

If the bully is acting out behaviour patterns learned in childhood, the same can sometimes be said of the victim. Randall describes a 'victim personality'. Care must be taken not to assume that any degree of blame lies with the victim, but there are personality traits such as timidity, low self-esteem and submissiveness, which make some people an easy target for the bully. Randall suggests the most common characteristics in victims of childhood bullying are insecurity, timidity, sensitivity, anxiety and cautiousness. It has been suggested that such victims have a tendency to cry more easily and attract attention to themselves in this way.

The 'classic passive, submissive victim' described by Randall, tries to placate the bully and shows no aggression. They make no significant attempts to win friendship, so they lack any peer support and appear isolated. This makes life easy for the bully who does not have to 'single out' a victim – the victim singles herself out. Bullying reinforces the victim's sense of low self-esteem and confirms their tendency to social withdrawal.

Once established in childhood, Randall asserts that the victim may continue such behaviour into adulthood, possibly remaining a 'loner' with poor social skills and little or no peer support. This then makes them liable to become a victim of workplace bullying too. However, we must stress that social skills can be learnt at any stage in life, and this is an important point to remember when assessing or mentoring an individual who may need to develop these skills further.

It is important to emphasise that many of the character traits assigned to Randall's 'classic' victim are also associated with certain illnesses such as depression. Childhood depression was a previously unheard of condition and even now is only just beginning to be researched. It is also possible for a previously gregarious, outgoing person to become temporarily withdrawn. Even during a temporary phase this person could become a victim of workplace bullying which could make recovery from their illness a protracted affair.

Care must be taken then not to assume 'once a victim always a victim'. Any of us could become the target of a workplace bully, which is why initiatives should be in place to protect all of us from workplace bullying. This extract from the 1994 MSF conference sums up this point quite effectively:

Interaction Between Individuals

Bullying was seen as a process of interplay between factors residing in the bully and the victim. It was important to understand this because the victim needs to see that he/she is not defined as 'a victim' any more than the bully is defined as 'a bully' in some immutable way. The victim needed to be clear that there was no question of blame, and needed also to be discouraged in every possible way that there was a hint of personal blame for the experience he or she had suffered. Understanding why the bully behaved as he/she did, could also help the individual bullied, to reclaim a sense of power and control. (MSF, 1994)

Male and female bullying styles

As with language and attribution style, there is also a significant gender difference in the style of bullying likely to be adopted. Men tend to adopt 'rational' bullying behaviours: that is, there appears to be a rational basis for their behaviour. Women, on the other hand, tend to use social manipulation whereby colleagues are used to act in an aversive manner towards the victim. This fact was reflected in the RCM study (1996) in the styles of bullying reported by midwives, and is aptly illustrated in the case study earlier in this chapter.

Language and Communication

Accurate assessment of a perceived threat is key to survival. Verbal threats can be direct but even veiled threats are still perceived as such. In the absence of a direct threat, language can still be perceived as threatening by virtue of the tone or content. It has been suggested recently that only 7 per cent of what we perceive from what people tell us is verbal, whilst 38 per cent is derived from paralinguistics (Paralinguistics: style, manner, tone, medium) and 55 per cent is from body language (*The Observer*, August 30, 1998).

Language and non-verbal communication are the media through which female bullying is dispensed. Interestingly, during the authors' research for this book, and earlier work, many of the female nurses and midwives did not use the term 'bullying', but instead claimed they were harassed, 'sent to coventry', 'had promotion blocked', their 'work was devalued' or they 'didn't get credit'. It seems that in the past, behaviour has only been considered as bullying when it involves overt physical bullying of the male style.

As mentioned above, female bullying adopts a different approach which is covert and manipulative but no less harmful: possibly more so because of the occult nature of the traumatic events involved. The trauma can be prolonged over many years before the bullying is discovered and addressed, possibly because the victim herself may not notice that something is happening until she starts to develop symptoms and wonders why she isn't 'coping' as she used to. By the time symptoms such as depression develop, the psychological damage has been done.

This form of bullying is all the more powerful when used by women against women, because of women's need to use language and paralinguistics in order to network. According to Tannen (1992), networking is the most important way women form relationships and become inaugurated into a community. Language is the most important factor in the development of these networks. There is increasing research on the importance of the use of language in networking and forming loyalty ties. Though women have the edge in this area, men are catching up fast. Researchers from vastly differing fields are coming to amazingly similar conclusions.

Tannen's work highlights how men and women use conversations for different reasons, but ultimately those reasons have an impact on social standing. Interestingly enough, Dunbar (1996) arrives at the same conclusion though his work is with apes and his theories centre around the evolution of language. Ultimately it looks as though our conversations, language and paralinguistics serve solely to either make or break loyalty ties. Once this is understood, the power of language, and its particular importance in female bullying, becomes apparent.

> A *sharp tongue is the only edged tool that grows keener with constant use.* (Washington Irving, *Rip Van Winkle*)

Body language

Morris (1989) suggests there are observable behaviour variables which warn of 'aroused aggression' and form part of the communicative process which is collectively termed body language. Morris describes insult signals, which are ways to show disrespect and contempt, which he differentiates from threat signals, which are aggressive in nature and are used to intimidate without coming to blows. According to Morris, threat signals, such as fist-shaking, are never misinterpreted.

This is possibly more pertinent to the male style of bullying, though one of the authors was once intimidated by a female senior midwife who had shaken her fist and thumped it down on a desk. This was an obvious threat signal which the author involved immediately perceived as unequivocally intimidating! Morris (1989) describes this action as a Vacuum Gesture: a stylised punch can be thrown, without touching the victim's body, but the interpretation is the same and the effect on the recipient is one of fear of future violence.

Neuro-linguistic programming

We want to briefly mention Neuro-Linguistic Programming (NLP) because of its current popularity in management training, though it is too large a topic to cover in depth here. The term NLP may be familiar to those in general management and especially in the field of Human Resource Development, but will probably be unfamiliar to nurses and midwives. NLP can be thought of as the practical application of many of the previously mentioned psychological theories. The originators, John Grinder and Richard Bandler, were a linguist and a mathematician respectively, but they studied the work of early therapists such as Milton Erickson, Fritz Perls and Virginia Satir. They were interested specifically in which psychological techniques could bring about change. NLP is often therefore resorted to when considering change, either in oneself or one's organisation.

As with comparisons between Tannen's work and Dunbar's, we often come across a phenomenon being researched by scientists from differing disciplines and the particular phenomenon under study is often accorded a different name, depending upon the professional language applied.

This is also the case with NLP. Many parallels can be seen with other psychological theories, but with NLP the difference is that it focuses on the practical application of theory specifically to bring about positive change, enhanced performance and the achievement of excellence (results) in business.

NLP is quite complicated and packed with jargon, but the principle is to focus on what works: focus on that which is excellent and what 'excellent people' (i.e. experts or masters in their field) do. It claims to be able to turn people into successful leaders by modifying their behaviour. NLP is currently enjoying a surge of popularity amongst managers because of these promised benefits.

> It is a way of coding and reproducing excellence that enables you consistently to achieve the results that you want both for yourself and your business. (Knight, 1995)

The interesting point about NLP, and the reason why we have included it here, is that the rise in the popularity of NLP in management is bringing with it a change in management culture. Many managers now believe that measurable change at a personal level is possible, in contrast with the outmoded belief that 'a leopard cannot change its spots'. Managers now value the importance of good communication, involve the workforce in organisational change and understand the importance of good staff support. Communication is the key to learning: a communicating organisation is a developing organisation. Managers who study NLP are more likely to desire to be charismatic leaders, communicate well and are less likely to resort to bullying their workforce to achieve results. Moreover they are more likely to understand the importance of coaching (mentoring) in employee development (see Chapter 7), which is that effective coaching can, and does, result in cultural change within an organisation.

> *The business world is changing so rapidly that the need for expertise in specialist skills has been replaced by the need to learn and differentiate.* (Knight, 1995)

Transactional analysis

In contrast to NLP, Harris (1973) also describes a process by which previous emotional experiences and feelings about oneself can permeate and influence social interactions.

Harris uses the concept of 'OK-ness' (sic) to explain whether people feel 'OK' about themselves and others. He suggests an 'I'm OK – you're OK' transaction as the most developed and the one to which people should aspire. He suggests that the majority of people display a 'I'm not OK – you're OK' emotional response which reveals underlying insecurity, and the belief that others are better than oneself.

Harris argues that where children have been physically abused they develop an 'I'm OK – you're not OK' attitude which stays with them throughout adulthood. This denotes an attitude of self-trust and a hatred for all others. Harris suggests this attitude is present in 'incorrigible criminals' who believe they are OK no matter what they do and that any concept of blame always exists externally – with others. Harris concludes by suggesting the ultimate expression of this attitude is homicide where the killer feels justified because he is convinced he is always right in all situations.

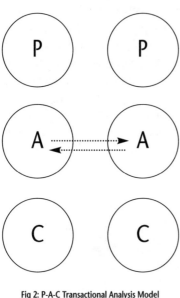

Fig 2: P-A-C Transactional Analysis Model
an adult-adult transaction

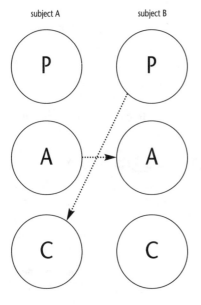

Fig 3: P-A-C Transactional Analysis Model
a crossed transaction

Harris uses Berne's (1964) transactional analysis model to illustrate the complex ways in which transactions can be intended and received. Everyone has within them a Parent, an Adult and a Child which, according to Harris, are not roles but a 'psychological reality'. Because of past experience and learned emotional responses, we may use any of these three in a transaction. For example, Harris gives a patient-nurse transaction:

> *Patient:*
> *'I would like to work in a hospital like this.'*
>
> *Nurse:*
> *'You can't cope with your own problems.'*
> (Harris, 1973)

Harris gives this as an example of a crossed transaction: the patient spoke as 'Adult to Adult', but the nurse responded as 'Parent to Child'. In this example the patient would have interpreted this response as patronising. Harris also discusses concepts such as 'angry child' or 'angry parent'. If one initiates an Adult to Adult transaction expecting an Adult to Adult response (Figure 2), yet the other person responds as 'angry' parent (Figure 3) or child , one could perceive this as intimidating. The stimulus for such a response may have nothing to do with the initiator, or the context of the interaction, but may be due to learned emotional responses within that individual.

Chapter 4

The effects of bullying

Bullying renders the victim impotent:
fear paralyses.

Ruth Hadikin

In view of the nature of psychological harm evidence is, often out of necessity, subjective and anecdotal. It is therefore not possible to establish unequivocal cause and effect. However, despite the reservations of the medical profession, this does not reduce its validity in the view of wider society, the 'victim', and (as will be examined later) British law. It has been suggested (Adams, 1992; Field, 1996; RCM, 1996) that workplace bullying is associated with increased stress and stress-related disorders, high blood pressure, alcoholism, anxiety disorders, gastrointestinal disorders, depression, post traumatic stress disorder and suicide. It appears that conditions such as workplace stress are multi-factorial in origin and in their effect on the individual.

Though in this section we refer predominantly to examples within the midwifery profession (as this is the area we have researched) the effects are analogous with many service industries where staff are in direct contact with the public, such as nursing, teaching and social work. In such areas the effects of workplace stress are compounded.

In a recent article on psychotoxic working environments, twelve workplace stressors were identified. These were:

- Unrelieved task overload, high pressure
- Needlessly intimidating supervision, rule by fear
- Bullying, discrimination, harassment
- Monotony, boredom, under-used capabilities
- Little control and low decision-making influence
- Changes: even those meant to humanise and improve conditions: being shunted around
- Ambiguous roles, blurred lines of authority
- Conflicts, not getting along with supervisors, work mates
- Social isolation, lack of support, poor communication
- No feedback, lack of encouragement
- Few learning, career or promotional opportunities
- Competition and job insecurity

Source: The psychotoxic workplace: Tracking job stressors. (An Internet document, http://www.convoke.com/markjr/toxic.html)

High pressure and low control: a deadly combination

We were able to apply between 9 and 12 of these factors to the situations of the midwives who wrote in to us. High pressure and low control are the two main stressors to which most midwives are subjected, and yet in our research and in the RCM survey, even midwives themselves did not recognise it.

> *Unremitting job demands, coupled with little or no control, can grind people into the ground. The combination is a deadly duo that produces not only mental strain, but can also elevate blood pressure and increase heart disease risks. Authoritarian practices that allow employees little or no influence over the pace and execution of tasks produce great distress.*
> Source: The psychotoxic workplace: Tracking job stressors.
> (An Internet document, URL: Http://www.convoke.com/markjr/toxic.html)

This was also supported by the Sheffield study (see later in this chapter).

Bullying in the workplace has an effect like dropping a stone into a pond. There are the effects on the individual concerned but there are also wider effects on the NHS in general. Staff can witness repeated bullying and may be living in fear of, if not directly experiencing, bullying. There are effects on clients and students. Nobody is comfortable working with a bully.

Quine (1999) found that 42% of people in her study had witnessed the bullying of others and that most of this witnessing occurred when the employee was new to the organisation and hence more vulnerable and less likely to challenge it.

As mentioned earlier, it is a feature of the human condition that the majority of people in new surroundings or with a new cohort first observe the accepted behaviour, dress, mannerisms and speech patterns and hierarchy of the group whilst on the fringe of the group. To be accepted by the group the newcomer has to quickly prove that she understands the culture and accepts it. In the NHS there are rituals that may occur around manner of speech, tea breaks, and attitude to other groups of staff. (For further reading on 'tea-break rituals', see Hunt & Symonds, 1995.)

The more quickly the newcomer embraces these norms of attitude and behaviour, the easier his life in the organisation becomes. It is often easier to become part of the culture than to fight the system. If this includes observing bullying behaviour and either copying or condoning it by not reacting, commenting or reporting it then the culture of bullying will persist. The effect on the individual could be that they too will become part of the bullying culture or, if they speak out, may be in danger of becoming the focus for the bully's attention, or have to leave that department or NHS Trust. It is easy to see that the organisational culture which condones bullying is self-perpetuating.

Case study

It was only when I left midwifery I realised what a monster I had become. By not doing anything I had become one of them. I should have spoken out well before Doris committed suicide, as I had watched her being pushed and pushed by the set of midwives whose aim was to make her miserable. We knew nothing about her except that she wasn't like one of us and didn't fit in. We all thought that work would be better if she wasn't there, but no-one thought of her at all. I feel so guilty that I was part of the game that had such disastrous results. No one ever talked kindly to Doris or tried to get to know her so we didn't know anything about her home life, where she trained or anything really. She was just different and took all the nasty comments, silences and exclusions from the group as though she didn't care. Although I didn't think of myself as one of the bullies I did nothing to stop it even though deep down I knew it wasn't right. I should have spoken out or at least been kinder to Doris. Now I will have her death on my conscience till I die. I feel ashamed of myself, but they [the bullies] feel no remorse and are still carrying on the same way.

Further research is necessary. For example, do we know what the effects will be on people who witness bullying though they are not bullied?

Case study

There was something horrible in the department but whether it came from the manager or the midwives I don't know. There seemed to be a lot of gossip and everyone seemed to try to get one over on each other. I couldn't identify who was friends or enemies with who and decided that the best thing to do was not to gossip, just listen. Eventually I did identify that large scale and long term bullying was going on, starting with the manager and her chosen few, and the bullied then became bullies to those who were under them and so on. It was a very unhappy place and I didn't stay long. As soon as I could, I got another job and left. As far as I know it is still going on and all anyone does is complain that they hate working there.

The cost of bullying

From these direct quotes from letters we have received, it can be seen that not only the victim but individuals and organisations can be affected by a bullying culture or by individual bullies. The effects are far reaching and the bottom line is twofold:

Bullying is costly to the organisation in time, money, personnel, recruitment and retention

and

Bullying affects patient/client care by rapid staff turnover, stress amongst staff and unhappiness of the staff that affects their commitment and kind caring.

Direct monetary costs can arise from legal action:

...in a recent case, £100,000 was accepted in an out-of-court settlement by a teacher who alleged that he had been bullied by the head teacher and other staff. (Dimond, 1999)

There are now precedents in British law whereby employees have taken an employer to court, specifically in relation to workplace bullying. The legal aspects will be considered in the following chapter. The human cost is related to the effects of the stress associated with workplace bullying.

Effects of stress

Griffiths (1981) describes stress as:

being driven beyond his [sic] powers of coping... beyond some optimum at which he [sic] can function most effectively.

This definition contains two elements which are important. These are:

the concept of being driven by some external person or factor which, importantly, one feels is beyond one's control, and that one's ability to function effectively will be compromised.

This reflects the powerlessness and impaired function described by many of the midwives who contacted us. Griffiths claims that the effects of stress can involve disorganisation which may present as inefficient problem-solving and/or the breakdown of skilled behaviour.

There are important implications for the NHS if essential, highly skilled professionals such as doctors, nurses, midwives, radiographers and all the allied professions suffer from inefficient problem-solving and breakdown of skilled behaviour, or even disorganised behaviour. How many of us work with people who could be suffering these symptoms, yet we just assume they are 'dizzy', lacking concentration, suffering from pre-menstrual tension or going through the menopause?

The rise in litigation, formal complaints and misconduct could be related to the effects of stress and the feeling of being pushed beyond the limits of coping. The effects of changing work and management practices that occurred during the 1980s and 90s have also been contributory to the amounts of stress being reported. (See research from Sheffield later in this chapter). Powerlessness in one area can result in over use of power in another area.

In areas where lack of control has been a key factor, staff can also demonstrate a learned helplessness which can carry over into their everyday lives. In midwifery, it has been suggested that work-related stress is linked to burnout and that the effects of this can be minimised by social support (Sandall, 1997). Bakker et al (1996) found that, among Dutch midwives, emotional exhaustion linked to burnout occurs less frequently in those who adopt an active coping style and more frequently in those who adopted a passive coping style.

Bakal (1979) claims that depression can result from an existential neurosis resulting from repeated attacks by others on one's core beliefs and values. Existential neurosis has been described as meaninglessness or

... chronic inability to believe the truth, importance, usefulness, or interest value of any of the things one is engaged in or can imagine doing. (Bakal, 1979)

Bakal explains that individuals such as doctors and nurses, who define themselves solely in terms of social roles and biological needs, are prone to develop an existential syndrome. Such individuals are inclined to worry whether others view them as conscientious or 'a nice person'; the expressed disapproval of others has a powerfully negative effect. This fact is supported by research (RCM, 1996; MSF, 1994) which shows that people become depressed when core values relating to their self, work or practice are constantly and repeatedly challenged by a bully.

The effects and incidence of stress among staff in NHS Trusts was the subject of a report undertaken by the Institute of Work Psychology at the University of Sheffield and the Psychological Therapies Research Centre at the University of Leeds by Borrill et al between 1994-1996 and 1996-1998. The research was a large-scale study funded by the Mental Health of the NHS Workforce component of the NHS research and development programme on mental health. It was based on data from two samples of over 11000 respondents taken in two time based samples. The study looked at:

● Levels of stress amongst employees in NHS Trusts

● Work factors associated with stress

● The relationship of stress with sickness and absence

● The effectiveness of selected interventions in reducing stress.

Copies of the full report can be obtained from Nicky Wheeler on 0114 222 3266 for a small charge.

We felt that quoting the main findings of this research would be useful to inform readers of the width and depth of stress within NHS Trusts.

Levels of stress among employees in the NHS:

1 *The overall percentage of people suffering from significant levels of stress was 26.8% in 1996 and 26.6% in 1998.*

2 *The level of stress remained very stable over time for the samples as a whole as well as for different occupational groups (i.e. managers, doctors, nurses, PAMs, P&T staff, administrative staff and ancillary staff) – with one exception.*

3 *The only occupational group to change was doctors, where the percentage of 'cases' decreased marginally from 27.8% in 1996 to 24.6% in 1998. This decrease is reported because it reflects a substantial change among junior women doctors.*

4 *There were considerable differences in stress between occupational groups, which were consistent over time. Managers recorded the highest proportion of 'cases' (33.6% and 32.8% in 1996 and 1998 respectively) and ancillary staff the lowest (20.4% and 23.1% respectively). In 1998 the level of stress for managers was significantly higher than for any other occupational health group except nurses.*

5 *The 'case' rate for NHS staff as a whole (26.6% in 1998) was considerably higher than that recorded among British employees more generally (18.4%).*

6 *Considering occupational groups separately, the NHS Trust managers had a 'case' rate more than 50% higher than managers in the general working population in both 1996 and 1998.*

7 *For nurses the 'case' rate was over 40% higher than for their comparison group (associate professional and technical occupations) in the general working population, again at both time points.*

8 *Doctors reported 'case' rates over 30% higher than their fellow professionals (e.g. lawyers, scientists) at both time points.*

9 *There was variation in stress across managerial categories. Junior managers and finance professionals had higher 'case' rates than middle and senior managers in 1998.*

10 *In 1998, women senior managers had much higher levels of stress than their male counterparts, the 'case' rates being 42.2% and 17.5% respectively.*
(Borrill, 1998)

These figures have been supported in varying degrees by all the research that we have studied for this book. They prove that stress exists at a much higher level within the NHS than in similar working environments outside. This is also supported by anecdotal evidence by people who have worked in both environments, and by the numbers of staff of all grades who choose to leave the NHS, not always for higher salaries.

The old phrase 'well, it's a stressful job', just isn't good enough anymore. In the light of contemporary research there is a lot more that can be done to reduce the stress of working in the NHS and make the NHS a healthier place to work. Tackling workplace bullying would be a major initiative in reducing stress in the NHS.

Work factors associated with stress, according to the research, were mainly:

> *high work demands, low influence over decision making, poor feedback on performance and high role conflict in both 1996 and 1998... Correspondingly, changes in work demands, role conflict, and influence over decisions, predicted change in employee stress levels between 1996 and 1998.*

Notice that the first two characteristics mentioned are the deadly twin stressors of 'high work demands' (high pressure) and 'low influence over decision making' (low control). The relationship between sickness absence and stress was proven in the research which stated:

> *Stress was related to absence. Staff defined as 'cases' reported twice as many days' absence in six months as staff who were 'non-cases' (5.2 days of absence in six months compared with 2.6 days). Correspondingly, staff defined as 'cases' had significantly higher rates of organisationally-recorded days absent for the six months after stress was measured (2.7 days compared with 1.6) than staff who were 'non-cases'. Self reported work performance was significantly worse for "cases" than for 'non-cases'.*

These figures are supported by local and national research into sickness and absence, and also by anecdotal evidence from our correspondents:

> *I just couldn't face seeing her [the bully] that I sometimes genuinely felt too ill to go to work but at other times I knew I could have worked but chose not to go in.*

> *My doctor was very supportive at first but I could tell that even he did not always believe my complaints... and neither did I. I*

just got very skilled in acting out the symptoms I had chosen... anything to avoid another day where I was made to feel inadequate and useless by X.

I knew exactly when I would come up against the tormentor and took steps to avoid those times. I felt really bad about not going in as my colleagues would have to do extra work but I felt so stressed by the thought of it that the symptoms of headaches and tension back pain were real to me.

The research also looked at different stress levels across NHS Trusts and found that they varied between 20.7% 'cases' to 31.5% . But there was no significant difference found when the research compared Community (NHS) trusts to teaching, or District General Hospital (NHS) trusts. They did find that the larger the NHS Trust, the greater were the levels of stress reported.

Two dimensions of climate were sufficient to explain trust differences... one was the extent to which training was emphasised and available and the other was the levels of co-operation and conflict.

This research successfully identified the levels of stress that employees felt they were under and the effect on work attendance patterns. It is more difficult to see from questionnaires that the effects of stress are caused and/or exacerbated by bullying. For this reason we must rely on subjective evidence from employees and anecdotal evidence. This form of research is often belittled by academics and is difficult to replicate. However just because bullying and its effects on the work force are unlikely to be charted or tabulated does not mean that it does not exist or should not be taken seriously.

The Sheffield research also attempted to identify interventions that may help to reduce stress in the NHS, and we will discuss these later. The first was that counselling services for those suffering from stress should be available, as this showed clear benefits for clients. They studied team working and their research showed that staff working in clearly defined teams reported less stress than their colleagues not in such teams. They put this down to the fact that being part of a team also gave social support (see Sandall, 1997) and they had clearly defined roles. Members of teams that achieved work interdependence and high team participation suffered from lower reported stress even up to eighteen months later.

In some cases, but not in all, an intervention following feedback on management styles by staff to their managers resulted in improvements. This appeared to be dependent on the level of commitment by those involved. However two larger scale interventions, which introduced 'Programmes of Care' and 'Stress Workshops', had no demonstrable effect on those who reported stress.

From this highly respected research we can deduce that staff stress needs organisational intervention and nowhere more than when bullying is a direct or indirect cause of stress. It does however come through the report that it is difficult to sustain these initiatives. Some areas that militate against sustained success in reducing stress were:

- lack of sustained management support
- lack of a clear overall strategy
- insufficient employee involvement
- an organisational culture which is not consistent with an emphasis on employee mental health.

This seems to support other information from many sources, even going back to Florence Nightingale's saying that 'hospitals should do the patient no harm', which in this context could be altered to: 'the NHS should do its staff no harm.'

Muriel O'Driscoll, who has lectured extensively on the subject of stress, often suggests that the 1980s and 90s management-jargon used by NHS Trusts, 'mind over matter' could be altered to 'we don't mind and you don't matter!'

One could argue that as victims of workplace bullying become more depressed, and thus more likely to feel powerless and self-blaming, they are likely to become locked into a cycle of abuse. It is important for victims of bullying to recognise that the fault is not theirs. Indeed, it is important that victims themselves recognise that they are being bullied and that this does not arise from some inner failing. If the victim does not realise they are being bullied they may inadvertently be supplying the bully with reinforcement that their bullying behaviour achieves results:

I remember working more than my allocated hours, always willing to help out, assist others and always put the students first. I was involved in various university committees, wrote articles, completed a Masters degree without a thought to the effect that this was having on my family or my health. I suppose that at the back of my mind I was trying to make myself indispensable... sometimes one is too close to realise that one is a victim. (O'Driscoll, 1997)

During research for this book it became clear that both the midwifery profession, and individual midwives, were seen by clients to be in a position of authority. Indeed midwives do have formal authority. Yet this is in stark contrast to some midwives' perceptions of their own position. The midwives who wrote to us felt they had little or no control and that they were over-supervised.

In the context of midwifery supervision, whilst outdated and ineffective practices must be challenged, consideration should be given to the appropriate environment.

Case study

Carol, a Staff Midwife, was accused of a drug administration error. One morning she received a letter informing her that she was to attend a disciplinary hearing to address the allegation. However, before this hearing took place, Carol was invited into the manager's office where she claims she was intimidated into making a 'false' confession. The Midwifery Manager suggested to Carol that, to avoid the stress of a formal disciplinary hearing, if she just owned up to the error the matter could be dismissed. Unwisely, Carol agreed and thought that would be the end of the matter.

When Carol next turned up for duty she was informed that she was 'on supervised practice'. This had not been mentioned at the meeting with her manager. The matter had not been dismissed; far from it. The whole department now thought her professional competence was questionable. She felt humiliated and betrayed.

Disciplinary hearings are indeed stressful, formal, situations but Carol would have had the opportunity to answer to the charges made against her. In this way she could have cleared her name and kept her professional reputation intact. Instead, she was bullied into making a false confession which damaged her reputation and allowed her professional competence to be questioned.

Carol unwisely accepted blame for an error which she believed she did not make. One could argue that this response was the result of a tendency towards self-blame, exacerbated by the intimidating confrontation with the manager, in the context of her perception that events were beyond her control. However, one could also suggest that Carol was challenged in a wholly inappropriate, if not bullying, situation which was specifically intended to intimidate her. Her reaction to the intimidating incident resulted in her poor decision-making as an attempt to end her immediate discomfort. This was in spite of her belief that she had not, in fact, made an error. This example illustrates the power of intimidation especially, as in the above example, when the abuser is in a position of authority. Bullying renders the victim powerless: fear paralyses.

The above example also raises issues about how we treat each other as professionals when we do make an error. If we cannot discuss practice in a safe environment without feeling that we are to be the subject of a witch-hunt, then inappropriate or out of date practice is likely to persist. As professionals, we need an open forum where we can debate practice. Are we incapable of helping colleagues and ourselves to keep up to date without apportioning blame? Whilst recognising the need to ensure public safety, the threat of professional incompetence has for too long been used as a stick with which to beat unpopular colleagues. Over-supervision without adequate support systems only contributes to job stress, and the fear of retribution increases poor decision-making and hence increases the likelihood that staff will make mistakes.

There is also the question of whether midwifery, in particular, is over-supervised and under-supported. In any context where a group is given a policing role, there should be structures in place to avoid an abuse of that role. Who polices the police? In our research, bullying by Supervisors of Midwives was, thankfully, rare but on the occasions when it was reported to us (as also mentioned in Chapter 1) it had a particularly powerful and damaging effect on the victim, who was left without any peer support whatsoever.

In a profession where communication, co-operation and support from colleagues is essential to one's ability to perform well, the withdrawal or denial of these can reduce one's professional competence. Nurses and midwives rarely work in isolation; peer support, in addition to mere co-operation, is often essential to good practice. Bullying can therefore have serious implications in our profession. Once one's reputation is damaged it is difficult to repair and, if a bully is determined to make one appear incompetent, colleagues may view one with suspicion for a long time thereafter. It is often necessary for a victim of bullying to move to a different department, if not to a different hospital, in order to regain respect and trust from colleagues.

It may be that the UKCC requirements for clinical supervision can function as a safety valve to allow nurses and midwives to explore interpersonal support and difficulties within the team. In some hospital and community areas, clinical supervision has been redefined, and 'clinical support groups' remove the hierarchical approach that can be at the root of further abuse. One of the key concepts of clinical supervision or support is safety to speak out without fear of reprisals in order to improve the level of service and care for the client. Like many good ideas this can be abused if the perpetrator of harassment is in a powerful enough position to influence the development of clinical supervision, and then the whole system simply reinforces the existing problems instead of attempting to solve them.

In midwifery, the role of the statutory Supervisor of Midwives can be used to good effect. Supervisors are now required to undergo an initial training and education programme with regular updates to enable them to fulfil the requirements of the role. These include the ability to support a number of midwives and to be a colleague, counsellor and advisor, and to promote a positive working relationship which is conducive to maintaining and improving standards of practice and care.

The potential for intimidating behaviour within the work environment to exacerbate an already stressful situation, resulting in ineffective, irrational and potentially dangerous behaviour should be of particular concern to Midwifery Managers and Supervisors of Midwives. The fact that bullying increases sickness levels and staff turnover within a department raises issues for Human Resource Managers. Bullying behaviour can probably best be addressed within the context of the risk assessment strategy: the aim should be to reduce stress in the work environment and hence stress-related costs to the employer through sickness absence, recruitment and retention, and legal action from both service users and employees.

Bullying behaviour is linked with increased alcohol intake (MSF, 1994). It is estimated that 10% of the workforce experience alcohol related problems; these people take an average of four times more sick leave than average, and at least 20% of accidents at work involve intoxicated people (Porteous, 1997). How much of this can be linked directly to bullying is uncertain, but in departments where bullying is a particular problem there may be indicators such as high staff turnover and abnormally high sickness levels which should alert management. The RCM (1996) study alone showed 15% of midwives claimed an increased use of tobacco or alcohol solely as a result of bullying.

Bullying has to be an issue of which modern managers are aware. It is no good pretending that it could not happen in your department, whilst wondering why your staff turnover or your sickness rate is so high. Care must be taken in using staff turnover alone as a guide to the general welfare of the workforce. One of the authors recalls a conversation with a Midwifery Manager who claimed that 'her' department was managed well because she had a low staff turnover. Bullying was rife in this particular unit, which was well known to one of the authors. Yet the manager was totally oblivious to the situation. She had failed to take account of the fact that an economic recession was preventing staff from leaving, as opportunities to move were reduced. Many midwives within the department were breadwinners, since their husbands and partners had become unemployed. The main indicator of a problem in this department was the excessively high sickness level.

Stress may be the result of being bullied, especially if this has been happening for a long time. It may also cause a person to use bullying behaviour in order to remain in control of an area of his/her life. This need to feel in control at work whilst feeling buffeted and manipulated at home is very common. It results in a strict adherence to rules, policies and procedures and an inability to be flexible. This can lead to a lack of tolerance for the actions of others and can also affect the client.

Case study

Mary was having a hard time at home. Her husband had been made redundant and now her earnings paid for the essentials, not for any extras. Her husband was becoming increasingly short-tempered and demanding, putting her down at every opportunity. Also, her latest smear report had shown that more investigations were needed. Although she chose not to discuss this with her husband or her colleagues she was worried about the long-term implications of both these events. Mary had never had a really close relationship with her colleagues but now she was unable to do anything other than give orders and insist on her standards being met. Eventually, she shouted at a colleague who reported her and a disciplinary interview was arranged. The midwife who had been on the receiving end of Mary's outburst made a statement and also asked the client to write to the consultant after the incident, which had 'ruined' the birth experience for her.

Far-reaching implications of bullying are not uncommon; invariably those affected ask the question 'how could this happen?' Ask yourself:

- Could this happen where I work?
- Do I know anyone who is behaving in this way?
- Is any member of my team or any associate displaying stress behaviours?
- What can I do to help, to listen, or to get them support?

The next example shows how long-term bullying can result in stress.

Case study

Sarah had been working on night duty for several years and did a steady job on the postnatal wards. Since the introduction of internal rotation to support team midwifery she now finds herself working in every department and often on day duty. On several occasions she has been publicly criticised and has felt humiliated by some of the other midwives. They now rarely speak to her and she feels ostracised by her colleagues. This has led to her feeling unhappy about coming to work, and fearful of making mistakes. It has affected her relationship with the mothers in her care and is making her suffer from insomnia, worry, headaches and depression.

In the both of the above cases the midwives would be horrified to be thought of as bullies, but that is what they are.

> Over 40% of charges faced by practitioners at Professional Conduct Committees involve some form of abuse, mainly physical and verbal (Source: UKCC, quoted from Midwives, Vol. 2 No. 2 Feb 1999 p.38)

The UKCC has produced guidelines on practitioner-client relationships and the prevention of abuse which state:

> the UKCC recognises that their [clients] needs will not be met while registered nurses, midwives and Health Visitors are themselves vulnerable to abuse within the workplace. All employers and health services managers are responsible for ensuring that practitioners can practise within the requirements of the UKCC's Code of Professional Conduct in an environment which is safe, supportive and free from abuse. (UKCC, 1999)

This responsibility of employers is discharged through employment law, and will be discussed in the next chapter. However, the message from the UKCC is clear: it is not possible to eradicate client abuse until we tackle and eradicate staff abuse, including bullying.

Bullying in midwifery education

If a bullying culture exists within the professional subculture of midwifery it is likely to be perpetuated through the educational system. Steinaker and Bell (1979) identified the following levels of experiential learning: exposure, participation, identification, internalisation and dissemination.

When students have followed different educational pathways, are educated to a higher academic standard and have different values and beliefs, why do they adopt the same subculture as older staff when they join a department? Contemporary research (Harris, 1995) has revealed some fascinating insights into this topic.

If one considers this issue solely in the context of attitude change alone, as discussed earlier, one can understand how students change their own attitudes to enable them to participate, identify and internalise the dominant culture. Indeed, when one considers this issue in the light of Harris' work, one can see they are forced to accept the dominant culture: failure to do so would result in ostracisation.

The special relationship between lecturers in higher education and the student midwife deserves special mention. Since the early 1990s nursing and midwifery education has been through a series of major changes with very little opportunity to evaluate these and adapt positively. From small local hospital-based training schools the education of future midwives and nurses was transported into higher education. This was done quickly and without the teachers having any control of their future. Higher education itself was also going through rapid changes as poly-technics became universities, colleges of further education were affiliated to universities and amalgamations of nursing/midwifery schools led to redundancies for some and rapid promotion for others.

At the same time, NHS Trusts were being set up, causing competition and secrecy instead of sharing and co-operation. Although the English National Board had produced a paper for 'Widening the entry gate to the professions', the universities were working to their own agenda of entry criteria. The academic status of the programme rapidly began to take precedent over the clinical and caring component. This in turn created extra stress for the teachers who were having to cope with a different culture, improve their own academic standing and also cope with being removed physically from the clinical environment and the support of their clinical colleagues.

Passing assignments became the main focus of activity for both teacher and student, sometimes to the detriment of the development of the individual student midwife. Academic rigour encouraged a more questioning and challenging approach to the subjects that older or earlier midwives had simply accepted. However, students were still expected to behave as 'empty vessels to be filled with knowledge', learning the trade of midwifery by copying the attitudes and even the speech patterns of their predecessors. Ingham and Fielding's (1985) work on the pressures to conform within institutions suggests that, despite a university education, contemporary midwifery students will still resort to 'traditional' practices (i.e. those of the dominant culture) on commencing hospital employment.

The fact that students attend an institute of higher education and an institute for midwifery practice placement means there is twice the opportunity for them to experience bullying. It has been suggested (Jowitt, 1997) that some students leave the midwifery profession solely as a result of the bullying which they have experienced. This has serious implications for recruitment and retention. In one institution in the North of England it was a frequent complaint that, at interview for admission to the course, applicants were questioned about their assertiveness, their ability to take responsibility for decision making, their communication and interpersonal skills and their ability to work within teams and individually. Yet students soon discovered that their lecturers treated them as imbeciles, failing to acknowledge their previous life and work experiences. This was repeated in the clinical situation in some instances. It seemed to the students that the greater their previous success and responsibility had been, the more the lecturers were determined to undermine them. The lecturers may have felt threatened as taking mature students with a more educated background was a new phenomenon in the 1990s. They were also trying to cope with new working experiences themselves.

Bullying or harassment can take many forms. One of these is to belittle and undermine the self-esteem of the individual through disregarding their contribution to discussions, allowing some students privileges but not others, and being unavailable for advice to some students. All of these have been documented more than once in letters from students to the authors.

Case study

Trisha, who had run her own business prior to entering midwifery, was reprimanded on her first day for asking about access to the lecturers for advice. She was told:

[lecturers] *were not there to spoon-feed the students and she must find out about things like everyone else.*

From then on she felt (and others in her group also noticed) that every contribution she made in class was ignored. She was also given her allocation at a centre 30 miles from her home, despite a more local student offering to change with her.

In cases like these the student must prove that the discrimination is only to the individual and be prepared to supply dates, times and witnesses for all instances. This is very rarely done and students, who are reliant on lecturers to pass or fail them, keep their heads down and do not complain through the correct channels or else decide that the pressures are too much for them and abandon the course.

Most universities now have anti-harassment policies, but the perceived power of midwifery lecturers is strong and student midwives rarely complain. Only when a whole intake of students agrees that bullying is a problem within the university is action taken. However, in the two cases reported to the authors the perpetrators are still in post and the complaints were put down to the

immaturity of the students

and

their expectations of the course being an easy ride.

The RCM (1996) study found that over half (109, 55%) of the respondents had considered leaving the midwifery profession because of bullying. The RCM surveyed qualified midwives. This does not reflect the wastage rate of students who do not make it as far as qualifying, though it is known that such rates are equally high if not higher. This high wastage rate of student midwives can have serious repercussions as the ex-students talk to their friends, acquaintances and their subsequent employers about their experiences as students. It does not take too long before the university department builds up a reputation of being unsupportive to students and applications and acceptances fall. This is especially true in areas where there is a choice of university to study midwifery. In some letters students have transferred to nursing courses as they perceive, incorrectly, bullying to be the preserve of midwifery alone.

An issue that may have had a significant effect on lecturing staff and added to their insecurity was the rapid amalgamation of small schools into bigger university departments with the subsequent threat of redundancy and loss of status. In midwifery the head of school was rarely a midwife and this resulted in a flat structure within midwifery education with little hope of progression. Added to this was the very real fear of redundancy and/or loss of status, with demotion for many. These circumstances do not excuse bullying behaviour but do give reasons for a lack of understanding and of support for colleagues and students.

Harassing an individual, perhaps to force a resignation, might take the form of allocating the only lecturer who does not drive and has to collect her daughter from the child-minder to the clinical area thirty miles away although other lecturers were willing to take the allocation. In a supportive team this could easily be discussed and the best solution put in place.

Where the team leader is threatened and unsure of the support of the team it is easier to stamp authority by giving orders without considering the whole picture. Some lecturers and midwife managers are so unsure of themselves that they see every innovative idea as a threat to their authority. They may sometimes take the idea and put it forward as their own. This is a common ploy of the bully as they are then in a win-win situation. If the idea is successful they take the credit. If it is a failure or not accepted they make sure that the instigator is then named, further undermining the victim's status within the organisation.

The shift from hospital to community means that more students have a relationship with one midwife who acts as their mentor and assessor. The intensity of such a close relationship would exacerbate the deleterious effects of bullying. The power that one person may have over another to first teach by example the caring role of the midwife and then to assess the student could be a minefield. The midwife may feel unsure of her knowledge base faced with a research-minded and well-read student. The midwife may also feel worried that the student is reporting to the lecturers on her standard of care and/or knowledge. This insecurity can result in the midwife being brusque with the student, and not encouraging questioning for fear of not being able to give a satisfactory answer.

This power differential within the relationship can lead to withholding of information, undermining confidence, putting the other person down at every opportunity, poking fun at their lack of knowledge, confidence or skills. If these ploys are used in the presence of mothers then the reputation of the whole profession can suffer. The student bullied in this way can soon lose what confidence she had and dread each interaction with the midwife. Her anxiety can affect her motor skills, making her clumsy and hesitant which, in turn, could place a mother and/or baby at risk. Students soon realise that some midwives are encouraging and supportive and others are less so. As students pass on such information both to each other and to the teaching staff this sometimes sets up a cycle of mistrust, dislike, avoidance and a very unhappy and unproductive workforce.

Problems such as this can be avoided by a good, supportive relationship between the college staff and the clinicians. Easily available updates for the midwives, covering assessment, clinical teaching methods and mentorship are essential, along with a close relationship between the school and the midwife and between the student and her support tutor. The worst scenarios that have been reported have occurred when there is a wide gulf between the school and the clinical areas, with both parties feeling stressed and failing to understand the problems and demands of each other's roles. Where a student feels 'got at' and undermined by both of the professionals who are supposed to assist in her clinical training and education, then there is a recipe for disaster.

The reputation of individuals is precious and can easily be destroyed by gossip, which can create a 'self fulfilling prophecy'. If a student or a midwife is reputed to be awkward, hard to please or withdrawn, then the reaction of those around her can make her behave in this way. Sometimes this reputation can be quite undeserved, with whole intakes of students being described by midwives and lecturers as 'the noisy group', 'the mad lot' or 'the quiet group'. Midwives may find themselves described as 'always helpful', 'not interested in teaching' or 'lazy', and wonder why they have to work harder to form a relationship with a new student.

Many education courses require the student and her clinical mentor to work closely together throughout the course. There is a certain amount of co-dependency in the relationship and many factors conspire to make it a success or a failure. The clinical midwife may see the student as the link with the education establishment. The student will take back reports to the lecturers about the midwife's skills, knowledge and attitudes and, if a bully is in place in the school this can have far reaching effects. We know of cases where midwives have failed to get onto a requested course simply because the senior lecturer has taken hearsay about her work from a student, and stored it away to be used against her in the future. This sort of power is rarely acknowledged, but does exist. The authors have been told of instances where the doors to further educational opportunities locally have been firmly shut for no good reason. This constitutes bullying or harassment, as one person is treated less fairly than another without good reason being given or indeed existing.

Case study

Sheila, a midwife, gave a student she was mentoring a fail grade clinical assessment. In the view of the lecturer, who had not worked with the student, this was unfair and she asked Sheila to change and upgrade her clinical assessment grade. Sheila was unwilling to do this as in her opinion the student had not reached competency in several areas of the assessment and a row ensued between the school and the clinical area. Sheila was eventually told that she was incompetent in assessment and was not allocated another student. Two years later when Sheila wished to register for degree modules, her application was refused by the same lecturer with no reason given. The implications of this type of insidious bullying are far reaching and there is very little opportunity to challenge decisions. Luckily Sheila was able to study for a degree by distance learning and she is well on the way to achieving her goals. In the process she has also been vocal in airing her grievances and dissuading other midwives from attending the local university.

This case illustrates the power of the student to act as a channel between the clinical midwives and the university. This can make life uncomfortable for the clinical midwife as she may try to hide her own perceived lack of 'book' knowledge from the student and give the wrong impression of her confidence. The midwife depends on the student for transmitting 'good reports' on her clinical work, teaching ability and attitude back to the lecturers.

The student relies on the midwife to demonstrate good practical skills, to discuss evidence based practice and to allow her to observe and sometimes copy her interpersonal skills. The midwife's approach to other people, in her attitude and spoken and body language, is also being noted, as are the midwife's approach and attitude to her profession, her employer, her manager and her role. All midwives sometimes hear, coming from their own mouths, the words of previous midwives they have known. These phrases and approaches are absorbed from our clinical teachers and are mostly of good quality and sensible. As mentioned earlier, this is how the midwifery culture is passed to each successive generation of midwives.

Most important to the student, though, is the clinical assessment. The clinical midwife/mentor is a powerful gate keeper and we have seen that power is a tool that can be misused or become a weapon. In the days when many Registered General Nurses (RGNs) followed on with midwifery training it was often the attitude of the midwife mentor that put them off staying in midwifery on qualification. In those days these people were not lost to the wider profession, as they usually returned to general nursing or went on to health visiting.

Today, student midwives who leave at the end of training or shortly after qualifying are lost to the health service and the expensive investment in their training cannot be recouped. Bullying attitudes are a significant factor in student wastage and recognising this fact and implementing strategies to remove or re-educate bullies should be a priority.

Midwifery is unique within the caring professions for having statutory supervision where each midwife is allocated a Supervisor of Midwives. Her role is to be a practising midwife and to maintain standards of practice, protect the public and act as friend, colleague, counsellor and advisor. She is the representative of the Local Supervising Authority. Generally this works well and is a mutually supportive arrangement. However, as mentioned earlier, there have been instances where this relationship has broken down due to bullying. In one area the unit manager was not only the Supervisor of Midwives but also the Regional Supervisor and this left the midwives who felt bullied with no support system at a local level. We will discuss later some of the measures that can be helpful in difficult situations such as this. Generally the Supervisor of Midwives is the first person to discuss a problem with but, as mentioned earlier, it is not unknown for Supervisors to be bullies.

Bullying can be a vicious circle:

> So, naturalists observe, a flea
> Hath smaller fleas that on him prey;
> And these have smaller fleas to bite 'em,
> And so proceed ad infinitum.
> (Jonathon Swift, 1667-1745)

The midwife who is being bullied sometimes retaliates by using similar behaviours with more junior colleagues, ward clerks, or ancillary staff. They may even bully women or their relatives. This was once accepted behaviour for ward staff as there were many rules and regulations to be insisted upon governing visiting times, mealtimes, sleep and bath times and even baby feeding times. Wards were very regimented places and the midwife was the metaphorical 'sergeant major'. In this context bullying was widely accepted as the chosen method of social control within institutions. Patients and their visitors were kept in place by making them feel uncomfortable within the ward. Nowadays there is a much more flexible routine within hospitals. With the development of a consumer society there has also been a cultural shift in attitudes towards healthcare. With people not only accepting more responsibility for their health but expecting it, when they do consult a healthcare professional they do so as a consumer and view the relationship as a professional consultation. They expect a professional discourse.

The bullying midwife may use other techniques to maintain her power, such as withholding knowledge and information from the mother and her family, deliberately undermining their self confidence and sometimes even giving incorrect information or instructions. This breakdown in the relationship between mother and midwife can have far reaching effects. For example, the mother may stop attending for antenatal checks, delay going into hospital or not report reduced fetal movements for fear of being ridiculed. This has been reported to us from across the UK, and we chose the following illustrative example.

Case study

Tracy was a drug addict, pregnant for the second time. Her first pregnancy had resulted in a stillborn baby at term plus 18 days. Since that delivery, within the same hospital, she had been made homeless, had become a registered heroin addict, had started on a methadone programme and was now living in a hostel. She was allocated a midwife working within a team who visited her at the hostel for her booking visit. Tracy would have preferred a hospital appointment for this visit as she felt quite ashamed of the way she was living. This comment brought the response:

We can't run our services round what you want.

The midwife never missed an opportunity to get a dig in about her lifestyle, fecklessness and lack of responsibility. Tracy began to dread the visits, and often made sure she was out when the midwife came to see her. Her social worker requested that Tracy's care could be given at the hospital but the midwife had already primed the Community Manager who stipulated that no 'special arrangements' were to be extended to Tracy.

This bullying behaviour towards an already vulnerable mother resulted in inadequate monitoring of the pregnancy, no relationship between the midwifery team and Tracy and no invitation to, or information given about, the services of parentcraft, aquanatal classes or other preparation for motherhood. The onset of labour saw a terrified mother, frightened to ask for anything in case she was 'told off', in fear not only of the midwife who had seen her but of all the staff that she met. The baby was small for dates and needed special care. Luckily the Special Care Baby Unit (SCBU) staff were able to overcome the damage done and by careful support and encouragement gradually increased Tracy's self confidence in her mothering skills.

A case conference was convened and the attitude of the first midwife was noted as she did her best to undermine the comments of the SCBU staff, the paediatrician, the social worker and the drugs outreach team. It was fortunate that this conference was chaired by an individual who recognised a bully who wanted complete power over Tracy and would stop at nothing to achieve her aim of undermining her by character assassination.

Although Tracy was especially vulnerable, all women, whilst pregnant, giving birth or post-natallly, are vulnerable. They are more emotional, their feelings are more attuned, they are more prone to weeping and they need the people and services to support them.

Childbirth and parenting is a new and unknown experience. It is a stressful time and no one behaves 'normally' when under stress. Many women play the role of wanting to please the midwife, to be a 'good patient' in order to gain the support and respect of the midwife. Where there is such lack of respect, or the midwife by expression, word or behaviour causes the woman to feel harassed, then the woman has grounds for a complaint of bullying, abuse or assault. Other situations of physical attack, during labour in particular, have been reported to us. Health professionals must understand that 'assault' in law is the fear of a physical attack and 'battery' can occur even when the client suffers physical contact without permission being given.

Chapter 5

The boss, the bully and the law

It is not necessary to prove that the defendant knew or ought to have known that his actions would amount to harassment

Halsbury's Statutes: editor's note to Section 1 of the [Protection from Harassment] Act, 1997

According to the Industrial Society, bullying costs the NHS money. Staff who are bullied at work could be costing their employers up to £200,000 in sick leave, redundancy, pension and other costs. A case reported in the *Liverpool Echo* on Tuesday July 6th 1999 quoted an £84,000 payout to a former council worker in an out-of-court settlement to compensate for years of bullying and harassment. The plaintiff had worked for the city council for eleven years as a domiciliary care manager before retiring due to ill health at the age of 51, two years previously. She was due to begin a claim for damages against the council for breach of duty of care. A spokesman of her trade union, Unison, said she had been subjected to harassment, bullying and intimidation for a number of years. She had complained about this through the council's procedures but they did not take any action, despite letters from her GP saying that her health was at risk and letters and reports from the council's own welfare and counselling advisor.

The spokesman said that she was forced to take early retirement because of ill health, and even then the council treated her badly.

> *They threatened court action against her for recovery of alleged overpayments while she was off ill. They also failed to honour a promise that she could take her grievances to a panel of councillors.*

The payment recognises the pain and suffering after years of ill treatment that she had to endure. Employers must be aware of such cases and take steps ensure that the workplace is as free as possible from bullying.

Although some cases will go through the civil courts with the 'victim' seeking damages, it is the employer who may well end up paying out through the vicarious liability offered to NHS and other employees. There are also manpower implications if legal proceedings are taken; not only may the organisation lose both the bully and the victim, but the bad publicity that ensues may make future recruitment difficult.

The Criminal Justice and Public Order Act 1994 (cited by Wells, 1997) makes it a criminal offence to intentionally cause harassment, alarm or distress to another person by the use of abusive or insulting words or behaviour, or disorderly behaviour. In addition to this, the 1997

Protection from Harassment Act (also cited by Wells) makes harassment on two occasions a criminal offence. This second act is especially useful as it targets harassment by name and although it is not specifically directed at the workplace there is no reason why it should not be applied in organisations. Under this Act a person can be convicted of harassment if he knows or ought to know that what he is doing amounts to harassment. Section 1 (2) of the Protection from Harassment Act states:

> For the purposes of this section, the person whose course of conduct is in question ought to know that it amounts to harassment of another if a reasonable person in possession of the same information would think the course of conduct amounted to harassment of the other.

The government did not list certain behaviours under this section because they did not want to limit the interpretation and extent of the term. The Act does expand on the sort of conduct which will constitute harassment as that which could include 'alarming the person or causing the person distress'. Harassment must 'involve conduct on at least two occasions'. The term 'conduct' can include speech. The intention, in describing harassment in this way, is to focus on the effect on the victim.

> It is not necessary to prove that the defendant knew or ought to have known that his actions would amount to harassment.
>
> (Halsbury's Statutes: editor's note to Section 1 of the [Protection from Harassment] Act, 1997)

This Act allows for both criminal and civil actions to be brought but actions could also be brought under the Disability Discrimination Act 1995, the Race Relations Act 1976 or the Sex Discrimination Act 1975 if the employee receives less favourable treatment on racial, disability or sexual grounds.

The legal position is shifting increasingly towards one where it is recognised that psychological damage can be inflicted by intimidating behaviour which may not necessarily include fear or threats of actual violence. Such behaviour in the workplace can either be considered a criminal offence under the jurisdiction of the 1997 anti-harassment legislation or, in the case of an isolated incident of intimidation, the plaintiff could allege criminal assault as a result of fear of harm.

The difficulty in such cases is one of evidence. Intimidating behaviour might, in the past, have been said to be largely a result of the victim's perception, but this excuse is losing credibility fast. The legislation is recent but it is only a matter of time before external indicators of intimidating behaviour will be legally defined as a result of precedent. The law has set precedents in the past by the application of old laws to new situations, as in the case of grievous bodily harm being extended to include psychiatric injury (Wells, 1997). Following the legal recognition of psychiatric injury, fear of violence can constitute grievous bodily harm as well as actual violence.

In considering the legal position on bullying we must not forget that some forms of bullying and discrimination have been acknowledged for years, as the Sex Discrimination Act (1975) and the Race Relations Act (1977) testify. These two Acts covered equality of treatment in employment, housing and healthcare. It could be argued that bullying on racial or sexual grounds has long been an accepted act within the health service and that people behave accordingly. Who knows how many people who challenge this behaviour are soon made to feel very uncomfortable and isolated?

Although the Acts are in place to support the individual, actually getting the evidence to take a case through the legal system is far from easy. Most people in this situation have spent months and even years being browbeaten and/or overlooked and may already be feeling insecure and with a poor self image. In cases of a widespread bullying culture, they will also lack confidence in the organisation's ability to address the issue, as demonstrated in the Stephen Lawrence enquiry (see Chapter 6). Their reserves of strength may have been so sadly depleted by the treatment they have received that they do not even apply for promotion or training courses, assuming that they would not be considered because of the underlying institutional racism or sexism that they know exists.

Case study

Florence had worked for the same hospital NHS Trust for many years as a State Enrolled Nurse on the postnatal ward at night. She was well thought of by the mothers, mainly because of her practical approach in helping the new mother to handle her baby. She had on several occasions asked for updating on breastfeeding practices and other topics within her sphere of practice, but had become used to having these requests ignored. Midwives who worked with her were always telling her that she was out of date and implying, if not saying, that this was her fault for not pursuing further education. Over several years, this attitude of other staff towards her became one of blame. Labelling Florence as lazy and uninterested in her work eventually became 'acceptable' amongst other team members and managers.

Despite her years of service with no complaints from her clients, when the hospital was due to close and transfer to a new building Florence found that her contract was not being renewed, due to her lack of educational advancement. Her manager actually quoted the gossip about her being uninterested in the work.

Florence had become so used to the attitude of her co-workers that she felt unable to challenge this. She was able to take up a post within the private sector where her talents and commitment were appreciated. Later she said that at her new job her first request for clinical updating was granted and she felt as though at last she was appreciated and accepted as an equal member of the nursing team. It was only when she left the NHS that she was able to recognise the bullying that had gone on.

Florence may well have been able to use the Race Relations Act to support her case had she wanted to take it further but, as in so many cases, the stress of complaining would have outweighed the stress of continuing. She had put in place her own individual coping strategies and also felt that in a white society managers and tribunal members would be likely to uphold the status quo. There seemed to be no value in going through the mechanism put in place by law.

This acceptance of the status quo, by large groups of employees, makes a change of attitude very difficult. Anyone who does complain, or act differently to their colleagues, could be perceived as challenging an institution that has stood the test of time, and risks ostracisation. It takes a very strong minded person to win a case and maintain respect from their colleagues and managers. In many instances it becomes a no-win situation: any satisfaction that may have been obtained through legal action can be offset by lost employment chances, lost friendships and damaged self-image. Financial payments are never sufficient to make up for the pain and the sense of loss.

The aforementioned Acts of Parliament are supported by several Codes of Practice which give guidance and state acceptable standards in various areas of life. The following are useful reference points:

- Code of Practice: Equal opportunities policies, procedures and practices in employment (Equal Opportunities Commission, 1985)

- Code of Practice on Sexual Harassment (European Community, 1991)

- Race Relations Code of Practice (Commission for Racial Equality, 1984)

- Code of Practice: Equality of opportunity in employment (Employment Equality Agency, 1983).

It is surprising how long these Codes and Acts have been in existence and yet how slow many major employers have been to put them into practice and to ensure that their employees are aware of the implications for the organisation. This does not just mean training for managers; awareness sessions should be provided by the training department and attendance should be compulsory. The benefits of these Codes to individuals must be stressed and the penalties of breaking the Codes must be made clear to every employee. The people at the top of the organisation must be seen to give serious consideration to incidents where equality of opportunity and treatment are not observed.

The Royal College of Midwives produced its own Equal Opportunities Policy in 1998, but many managers and RCM employees still do not know of its existence, let alone the general membership. Many employers will only change practice when forced to do so, which is the reason why Codes of Practice have to be supported by legislation.

The UKCC also supports equality of care by stating:

> [Each nurse, midwife or Health Visitor must] recognise and respect the uniqueness and dignity of each patient/client and respond to their need for care, irrespective of their ethnic origin, religious beliefs, personal attributes, the nature of their health problems or any other factor. (UKCC, 1992)

Whilst it is not stated that this applies to colleagues/employees as well as clients, it would be reasonable to expect that colleagues deserve the same respect. It is also states:

> [Each nurse, midwife and Health Visitor must] report to an appropriate person or authority where it appears that the health or safety of colleagues is at risk, as such circumstances may compromise standards of practice and care.

Many employees are in an excellent position to monitor the effect of harassment on their colleagues and can see the health and coping skills of the individual deteriorating, but do nothing to help to stop the bullying. This is easy to understand: to draw attention to it may make the bully turn her attention to them. There is also the unhelpful attitude that the victim somehow deserves the treatment they are getting, because they have failed to stand up to the bully as the observer may like to imagine that they would. This makes a division between those who are perceived to be 'strong' and those who are perceived to be 'weak'. Care professionals are almost by definition supposed to be 'strong' in order to care for others who are dependent on them, and the carer who is seen to be 'weak' is deemed not suitable for this demanding career.

The importance of recognising the effects of bullying and the subsequent stress caused to the individual is underestimated by NHS employers. Although the Protection from Harassment Act became law in 1997, few cases have been heard.

> A man was charged with using conduct in an NHS hospital which caused his victim to fear violence would be used against him and verbally abusing and threatening him between June and November 1997. (Source: Wirral Globe September 23 1998)

Bullying and harassment could be a disciplinary matter under an employee's contract of employment. This could raise the question of whether a single misdemeanour could result in criminal, professional (statute law) and civil (e.g. employer disciplinary) proceedings simultaneously. For example, will a bully be dismissed, struck off his or her professional register and receive a court sentence? Only the courts can answer this, but the most probable answer is 'No'. The reason for this is that the harassment law is not specific in this regard and is too easily open to interpretation. This argument is expanded in an article by Nick Reed LLB, LLM, DMS (*Stress News* July 1999 Vol. 11 No. 3). Here he states:

> *Under the Protection from Harassment Act 1997 will the 'reasonable person with the same knowledge as the harasser' be (notionally) someone who is employed in the same organisation as the alleged harasser? As the 'reasonable person' test is the one most likely to be used to determine whether particular conduct is or is not harassment, this would seem to be of some importance. Presumably, the sort of behaviour or conduct (particularly language!) which would amount clearly to harassment in a public library may well not qualify in the context of the Royal Marine Commandos.*

It would be helpful if legal proceedings could be avoided. Even when legal action is initiated it may help the employer if they can show that they have been aware of their responsibilities and have taken steps to lessen or remove harassment from the work environment. They must have in place (and well publicised to the staff and trade unions) documented evidence that such behaviour will not be tolerated, that complaints will be listened to and that appropriate action will be taken. Employers who have attempted to discover the extent of bullying as perceived by the staff working in their organisation will be better equipped to deal with the particular type of harassment within the culture of the organisation. There will be different types of behaviours which may be perceived as acceptable by some members of the organisation and not by workers or managers elsewhere. For example, nurses and midwives have in the past expected to be treated with little or no respect and given mundane tasks to do early in their career. Some even think that this is part of the initiation into nursing/midwifery and believe that it assists in the development and learning of the individual. For school leavers fresh into nursing this may have been the case as they learned to obey orders without question: a useful skill in an emergency! This can be compared to the bullying within the armed forces that produces the unquestioning, order-obeying soldier so necessary in times of conflict. However, where the mature entrant to the professions is given mindless and meaningless tasks at the whim of an authority figure, this may constitute bullying if the perpetrator is not consistent in this and is seen to favour one person over another.

Another recent Act that may be helpful to healthcare professionals in cases where they have in the past felt helpless to act is the Public Interest Disclosure Act 1999. The problems caused to employees prior to this Act being passed are documented in Chapter 6. Following a highly publicised case featuring Charge Nurse Graham Pink, and other cases, the nursing press and organisations began their 'whistle blowers' campaign.

The Act aims to protect the employee from victimisation or dismissal, and to protect the consumer from receiving less favourable treatment. In the past people who 'told tales' were considered disloyal to the organisation and their colleagues. However, there have been many high profile cases where inadequate, and in some cases criminal, treatment would not have come to light without inside information from the organisation or would have been discovered earlier if employees had felt safe to disclose information to the appropriate authorities. Public demand for more openness is also more evident especially after such disasters as the Bristol paediatric deaths, the cervical screening mistakes and the various 'misuse of public money' cases that have come to trial.

For the employee to have the legal protection that this law offers, any disclosure must be 'in good faith'; that is, the person must believe that it is true. It does not encourage or support vindictive or anonymous information. Some employees may not want to put their name to any complaint or inside information, despite the assurances of the Act. Inside informers should attempt to bring their concerns to the attention of NHS departments before going to the press or media. This may not necessarily mean within their own organisation if the problem is in danger of being covered up. It may mean involving the Health and Safety Executive, the Health Secretary or the Audit Commission, the government spending watchdog. Advice could also be obtained through the Community Health Council, from the Citizens Advice Bureau, or from the steward of a trade union or professional body.

During these initial stages of advice-seeking the informer can invoke anonymity for both themselves and the organisation or person being complained about. Confidentiality of client/patient details is of the utmost importance throughout the proceedings. Otherwise, in the case of nursing and midwifery, the employee may well set themselves up for investigation by the UKCC for not reaching the standards laid down in the Code of Professional Conduct. Only when all avenues have been explored and advice has been taken from informed sources should the employee go to the media. This must be seen as a last resort when it is felt that the matter is being covered up internally or organisationally and is still continuing.

Any employee can invoke the Act and it applies to part-time staff, agency staff and students. Some people may think that students would not be able to recognise malpractice or misuse of public funds, but newcomers often view the status quo with fresh eyes and before they have been immersed into the organisation's culture, can often bring a new critical perspective to a situation.

Mature students have often paid income tax for many years before entering the profession. They view the service from both the viewpoint of the consumer and the taxpayer. They are in an ideal position to evaluate how public money is being spent.

Employers and unions have welcomed this Act and many are working together to ensure that procedures are in place to enable staff to 'blow the whistle' safely. Malpractice can cost organisations millions of pounds in compensation payouts, recruiting and retaining staff and rebuilding a shattered reputation, so this opportunity to correct malpractice before great harm is done is to be welcomed.

In addition to the principles of common law outlined above, the midwifery and nursing professions are regulated by statute law. The relevant Act of Parliament is the Nurses, Midwives and Health Visitors Act 1979 and the midwife's legal responsibilities under this act are set out in the form of Statutory Instruments (UKCC, 1993).

Professional accountability

The Statutory Instruments (UKCC, 1993) clearly stipulate that each individual practitioner is personally accountable for his/her practice and that, in exercising this accountability, each midwife must safeguard the wellbeing of clients, ensure that no action or omission is detrimental to the client's safety and report circumstances where safe care cannot be provided.

In the following case study, the midwife is clearly guilty of professional misconduct as well as common assault. She could be removed from the professional register and could also be charged with grievous bodily harm. Her midwifery colleagues have a legal, professional and moral duty to report the incident.

Case study

Louise, aged 20, had hypertension at term. She was told labour would be induced. At 12 noon a doctor put up an intravenous drip and ruptured her membranes.

By 7pm she was in considerable pain, so she was given pethidine and transferred to a delivery room. She was alone. Her husband and mother were outside but were not allowed in. She says she was very frightened and didn't have a clue what was happening or how far on she was. She had wanted her mother with her.

She became aware of a midwife in the room. The midwife had her back to Louise and appeared to be busy. Louise doesn't remember her coming into the room and hadn't seen her before. She remembers moaning loudly with the pain and says:

...but I wasn't screaming.

The midwife turned around and suddenly slapped Louise across the face, saying:

Shut up. Don't be silly, you're only having a baby.

Louise says she will never forget it.

As a result of this experience she refused to have her second baby in hospital and still feels 'nervous of hospitals'. The above incident took place in 1970.

(This case study originally appeared in 'When Interpersonal Skills Fail' by Ruth Hadikin, *British Journal of Midwifery* 6:6, 366. It is reprinted with permission of the BJM.)

Some of the regulations that govern the work of midwives and Health Visitors can be misused by managers and employers. The regulations themselves can be used to threaten or over regulate the work of individuals. The following example shows how this can occur.

Case study

Sally was an experienced midwife working on a busy delivery suite. The whole department was understaffed and had recently been shaken by a new manager who had a more direct and demanding approach than the previous manager. The School of Midwifery had moved to the university and amalgamations within education meant that there was no longer any consistent support or advice from sympathetic and understanding midwifery teachers who were known to the clinical midwives.

On a very busy day, when Sally had been caring for three labouring women, she asked for help from the shift manager with one labouring woman, whilst she delivered one of her cases. When she returned to the first woman she found that her notes had been taken out and were being scrutinised by the manager and her colleague. She asked for them back so that she could continue her contemporaneous record-keeping in accordance with UKCC guidelines. At the end of her shift, with the women in her care all happily delivered of healthy babies, she was asked to account for her poor record-keeping. Sally said that she didn't think there was anything wrong with her notes, but the shift leader told her that they would be shown to her supervisor and to the Approved Midwife Teacher. These three people decided that Sally needed some updating and she was required to write a 3000 word essay on the importance of monitoring and keeping good records.

Sally felt that this exercise would not guarantee the expected outcome and that if she needed updating then a course or study day, or a practical exercise, would have been more use. When she mentioned this she was told that if she wanted to take it further then the UKCC would have to be informed and this would probably lead to her being disciplined or struck off. Several months later she overheard a student being told by the Midwife Teacher to 'watch her midwife' (Sally) as her record-keeping wasn't very good!

Sally eventually left midwifery. She felt victimised, and that the system of regulation had been misinterpreted. It seemed that no matter how well she did in midwifery this unsubstantiated complaint against her was not allowed to be forgotten.

Chapter 6

Acknowledging and altering a bullying workplace
Guidance for managers

We ask whether the workplace itself is to blame, stressful and competitive as it is, or are we all going too soft – encouraging people to see themselves as victims?

Joan Bakewell, *Heart of the Matter*, BBC 1, Sunday 21st February 1999.

Workplace bullying is viewed by some as a 'myth' which thrives in a modern society which has 'gone soft'. The topic is seen as controversial by the media and this possibly reflects the view of wider society. So do these views influence NHS managers in their approach to managing people?

During the BBC debate, whilst commenting on a specific incident, Ruth Lea (representing the Institute of Directors) said:

> It's not bullying... it's not persistent.

Whereas, as mentioned earlier (Chapter 3), Randall is clear on this point:

> Aggressive behaviour does not have to be regular or repeated for it to be bullying behaviour. (Randall, 1997)

Part of the problem, as mentioned earlier, is the difficulty of definition. Many managers still shy away from the term 'workplace bullying' because of the connotations with school bullying which managers find hard to conceptualise within a workplace situation. Managers often prefer to use the term harassment, yet it is this very association with harassment which leads managers to the belief that there must be a degree of persistence before a behaviour can be viewed as problematical or damaging to the workforce. Randall (1997) points to the inadequacy of the term harassment, in that it is limited in its ability to encompass other aspects of aggressive behaviour. Indeed aggression, and even violence, can occur as an isolated incident and it is not so much their persistence but the fear of a recurrence which leads to the psychological damage.

Whilst psychologists continue to debate whether behaviour has to be persistent, or intentional, and whether it should be defined as 'bullying', 'mobbing' or 'psychological terrorism', where does that leave managers and what, if anything, can managers do?

During the BBC debate Neil Crawford (psychotherapist and workplace consultant) appeared to be the voice of reason:

> When you're managing a complex task such as, for example, in the kitchens of top restaurants and you're having to deliver those meals, human relations go out of the window – and so it is in large organisations and the question for management is not 'how do I

get rid of it' but 'how do I manage that' because it's always going to happen. (Neil Crawford, *Heart of the Matter*, BBC 1, Sunday 21st February 1999.)

The various academic arguments over the definition of aggressive behaviour in the workplace might not hold much interest for managers. What should be of interest is the very real fact that such behaviour, regardless of how it is defined, can cost organisations dearly in hard, financial terms.

Case study – the John Walker case

In the early 1980s John Walker was leading four teams of social workers during a time when the workload was rapidly increasing. In 1986 he suffered a nervous breakdown and he did not return to work until 1987. His breakdown was attributed to increased levels of 'work related stress'.

On his return to work in early 1987 he was promised support from a Principal Fieldwork Officer which he got, but this was withdrawn as early as April that year. When he felt his levels of stress building up again he reported this to his employers who did not do anything about it. Consequently he suffered a second nervous breakdown and was dismissed by his employers on the grounds of permanent ill-health. He has since been unable to work in any post involving similar responsibility. Subsequently John Walker was awarded £200,000 damages in his case against Northumberland County Council.

During the court proceedings Mr Justice Coleman stated:

There is no logical reason why risk of psychiatric damage should be excluded from the scope of an employer's duty of care or from the coextensive implied term in the contract of employment. (Case Study adapted from Randall, 1997)

It can be seen that the court, in arriving at its decision to award damages, is less interested in academic descriptions of the behaviour which caused the psychiatric injury, than in the fact that the employer failed in its duty of care to the employee. In a sense it is obvious that certain aggressive and violent behaviours are likely to have a negative psychological impact on the recipient, regardless of which definition we use to describe such behaviour.

In Britain you call it bullying, in Sweden we call it mobbing but it doesn't really matter what you call it, the effects are the same. The word should really be replaced with psychological terrorisation.
(Klaus Klimer, cited by Andy Ellis in *Stress UK*, 1997, an Internet page.)

Given the difficulties in defining and identifying potentially harmful behaviours in the workplace, what can managers do to foresee and pre-empt claims of psychiatric injury? The focus for managers, in any anti-bullying initiative, has got to be on the concept of an employer's duty of care. A top-down approach is essential: employers must be seen not only to pay lip-service to the concept but to be demonstrably caring in their approach to the day-to-day running of the organisation.

Risk assessment

Organisations must make time and finances available to address bullying. A starting point is a strictly confidential questionnaire for all staff to complete, that defines bullying and harassment in its widest sense. The confidential aspect of this is essential. One NHS Trust decided to issue these questionnaires with everyone's pay slip, only to find that each person's employee number had been printed on the top of the questionnaire, making confidentiality impossible to ensure. Needless to say, the returns of that survey were minimal! Employers need to take steps to assess the extent of bullying, not only to prove that they have done so if an enquiry took place, or if they were the subject of legal proceedings in civil actions, but also to be able to identify what and where management action is needed to change the organisational culture.

Top-down approach: major change in organisational culture

Any major change within an organisation takes time, commitment and money. Organisational change, unless it is handled sensitively and professionally, can cause stress and upset to some, if not all, groups or individuals. To change the culture of an organisation requires a respected 'change agent' at the head of the organisation, someone who can persuade some, 'sell' to others and drag a few into the new and, hopefully better, culture of a bullying-free organisation.

Management structures and processes should be in place to enable cultural change and to facilitate the development of a positive working environment which would prevent 'old' behaviours from returning. There may well be casualties in this change and managers should be ready to transfer staff, to arrange for retraining or even to offer retirement/ redundancy packages for the few. However this should only be used as a last resort if development strategies have failed. Cultural change is challenging and painful as people have to give up what is familiar and comforting and confront unknown and untested feelings and emotions.

The I-A-B model for improving performance

Individual Performance Review (IPR) should be used positively to identify the level of development from which an individual employee might benefit. Where individual performance issues are identified, we suggest managers use the Information-Attitudes-Blocks (I-A-B) model (see Figure 4) as a tool in deciding what action would be most effective. At IPR interviews, if managers are confronted with an individual who displays problem behaviour such as bullying, there are three broad areas which can be explored to help target any management action: information, attitude and 'blocks'.

Does this person need information?

In other words, are they ignorant of their responsibilities, or lacking in skills? Would they benefit from further education and training? If so, refer them to an appropriate training course.

Have they got an 'attitude' problem?

Are they displaying attitudes and behaviours which offend others, such as racist language? Have they been on training courses which have not resulted in any measurable behaviour change? Such individuals are not always a lost cause. Referral to an external agency for assessment may reveal that they are 'coachable'. If the individual is deemed suitable, a period of coaching would result in the desired behaviour change. This is a win-win situation for both parties: the employee keeps her job, and the employer saves on the cost of dismissal and recruitment. With the expansion of coaching as a profession there is no longer any reason for employers to tolerate poorly performing staff. It is no longer a case of put up with them or dismiss them, there is a middle ground. Once coaching brings an individual back on-track, they may need additional training also.

Do they have personal problems which are 'blocking' their development at this time?

Temporary disorders, such as depression, can affect an individual's performance. The majority of people in this situation can recover provided they are supported and treated sensitively. They may then require some coaching and training to 'bring them up to speed'. The Occupational Health department is a great help in such situations, as can be Human Resource managers if, for example, an extension to the employment contract is required. Staff counsellors and professional therapists can be invaluable in identifying 'blocks' and helping the individual to overcome them.

Figure 4 shows that, within the I-A-B model, there are three main areas which must be addressed to facilitate change in an individual. People can move up or down between these areas. It must be acknowledged that in many cases it is not individuals but management processes which are at fault. Figure 5 shows how the employee development process works using the I-A-B model. Disciplinary action, and subsequent dismissal, are a last resort which would apply to very few employees. If an individual remains unchanged after counselling, coaching and training, one is lead to question why the individual was offered employment in the first instance and whether the organisation's recruitment strategy needs to be reconsidered.

The only way to turn around the widespread NHS bullying culture is through a major leadership initiative to orchestrate such change. A leadership-driven approach, initiated by government and implemented through the NHS Executive is the only strategy likely to have a lasting effect. Ultimately it is a change in attitude that is required: similar to the government initiatives to change attitudes towards drink-driving, a behaviour which was considered socially acceptable 40 years ago but is now considered deplorable. So it is with bullying. We are currently in a changing society in which we must stand firm and insist that this is deplorable behaviour. Government, NHS Executive, leaders, managers, colleagues and peers must all express their disapproval of such behaviour to effect a general change in attitude towards bullying. It must be seen and felt to be real and not just an exercise. The commitment to outlaw this behaviour must be explicit.

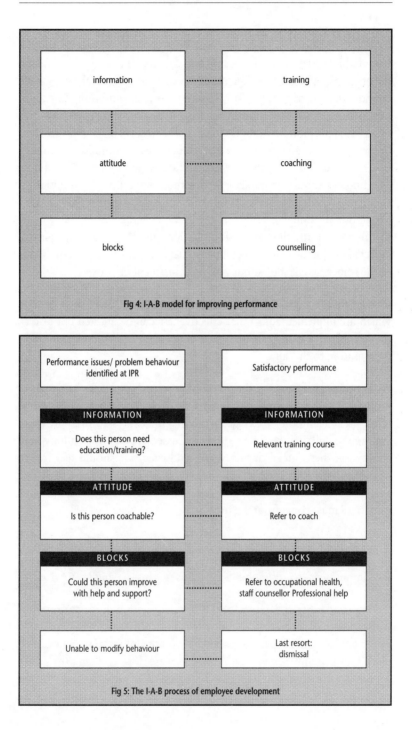

Fig 4: I-A-B model for improving performance

Fig 5: The I-A-B process of employee development

Disapproval of bullying should be explicit

It should be widely known that bullying will not be tolerated throughout the organisation. Staff-side organisations can be involved in the design and confidential distribution of questionnaires, in addition to policy formulation. Most importantly, agreement should be reached on which working definition to adopt. Since initiatives such as this are best originating from government, a government select committee would be best placed to look into the research and devise a nationwide definition. The findings should be implemented without hesitation. Such initiatives should be widely promoted to inform staff, with a government-funded promotional campaign involving television coverage as well as widely-distributed information packs. Information notices should be displayed, especially in public places so that consumers of the service are also aware of the stance taken, should bullying or harassment be proven.

Regular forums should be held to discuss the effectiveness of any initiatives which are implemented, so that effectiveness can be audited but also so that employees can be reassured of the consistency and commitment of the organisation to this aim.

As mentioned in chapter 2, the power of peers and colleagues in matters of attitude can never be underestimated. One of the key factors which would effect a change in the workplace would be the expressed disapproval of colleagues. Bullying should be openly discussed at every opportunity, staff forums, in the canteen during work, and everyone should feel free to openly express their disapproval for such behaviour. Victims of bullying will not feel in a position to initiate such discussions, which is why initiatives must come from the top.

Bullying must be specifically mentioned in harassment policies as 'gross misconduct', reinforcing the message that the organisation is serious in its commitment to erasing bullying and is not just paying lip-service.

Trying to identify the extent of the problem within an organisation is difficult, as the perception of bullying is quite different in the mind and experience of the perpetrator and the victim. Bullies may believe that since they are only doing the things that were done to them, this is not bullying. Identifying bullying or harassment is no easy task for the employer, as 'offensive' behaviour has to have a recipient who sees the behaviour as offensive and/or threatening, and is able to describe its effects on her life Although we acknowledge the very real difficulties employers have in identifying the extent of the problem in each work area, the fact that attempts have been made to identify the problem and strategies put in place to deal with it will certainly be in the employer's favour should a case be investigated or come to court.

Many surveys and questionnaires have been produced to assess the problems. These can often help to protect the employer by providing detailed data on perceptions of bullying, sickness and absenteeism, staff turnover, client satisfaction and so on. The data itself, however, cannot protect each worker from the behaviour of a minority of malevolent and often powerful people who make their victim's life a misery. The survey should always be seen as the essential first step in an integrated approach to the problem.

Another way of actively trying to determine the level of the problem is to include direct questions, either verbal or as a questionnaire, as part of a leaving or termination of employment interview held with departing employees. One hospital has taken the trouble to invest time and money by undertaking individual interviews with every member of staff. The aim is to try to identify perpetual bullies who are undermining the morale of the staff and hence affecting recruitment and retention of staff, and ultimately patient care. This could also be a part of existing interviews under the Individual Performance Review (IPR) system or, within midwifery, the annual review discussion between each midwife and her Supervisor.

Many organisations have now produced anti-harassment policies to try to address the problem. It must be stressed that for a policy to be effective it needs to be known by all members of the organisation and also needs to have punitive, as well as supportive, and manageable investigative powers. There should be involvement of union representatives in writing and reviewing these policies alongside management, personnel and worker representation. For a policy to be useful to the organisation, wide consultation and dissemination of the discussion is essential for it to be accepted and 'owned' by the workforce. There must also be a commitment from the highest level that recognises bullying as a serious offence.

Some employees will not complain of bullying for fear of further victimisation and this needs to be addressed within the policy. Well-publicised statements that bullying is unacceptable and will not be tolerated are useless if the employees perceive the management to be guilty of harassment. Confidentiality should be guaranteed until a formal complaint has been issued, and steps should then be taken to limit the opportunities for further victimisation.

Complaints (grievance) procedure

Complaints need to be handled speedily, sensitively and confidentially. These complaints must be treated separately from the normal grievance procedure which tends to be lengthy and often has to go through line management, which may be the main problem in bullying complaints. In the proactive organisation, grievance procedures would be designed to take account of the fact that the employee can have a valid grievance against more senior managers.

Most anti-harassment policies offer the choice of formal and informal procedures to follow and these two approaches can be used in either order. The informal approach could involve the use of specially trained counsellors with whom the victim can discuss what has happened and obtain help in deciding the best way forward. Where the first step in tackling the problem is to meet with the personnel department representative or a management-appointed person, the confidentiality component must be stressed. This initial contact may be with the trade union representative and again the opportunity for an informal approach should be stressed.

Some policies would allow for a note of the complaint and the outcomes of the discussion to be filed in a sealed envelope with the staff records of the person being complained about. This enables a consistent record to be kept with each person which will only be acted upon if a substantial number of complaints are received.

One disadvantage of this is that the complainer may feel that nothing is being done. It could also be used by a manipulative bully to work against the victim if follow-up investigations are not instigated.

A good example of this informal approach has been implemented by South Yorkshire Police. They define harassment as:

> *any unwanted or hostile or offensive act, expression or derogatory statement, including incitement to commit such behaviour, which causes distress or affects the dignity of men and women at work.*

Their 'First Contact' scheme is a confidential listening service to support those who have experienced racial, sexual or personal harassment. They seek to restore confidence, raise self-esteem and enable the complainer to pursue an informal or formal procedure. The options for informal procedures include:

- taking no further action but recording the complaint
- speaking to an equal opportunities advisor or personnel officer
- confronting the harasser
- considering external help.

Where confronting the harasser is chosen, this must be handled sensitively in order to protect both the complainant and the perceived bully. It can be done face to face with an advocate to ensure equality of opportunity for both parties to have their say and to finish with an agreed way forward. The aftermath of such meetings must be monitored in an agreed format and confidentiality for both parties must be maintained. It must be made clear to the bully:

- That their behaviour is contrary to the organisation's policy on bullying
- That their behaviour must change to comply with the organisation's expected standards
- What the impact of their behaviour is on their work colleagues
- That they must stop their bullying behaviour
- That the situation will be monitored
- What the consequences will be if the bullying continues
- That the discussion is informal and confidential at this stage.

The formal procedure can follow on from an informal complaint, or the victim may make it formal initially by putting the complaint in writing.

The anti-harassment policy must include a clear procedure to be followed and must also include a way for the complainant to bypass their manager where he/she is the subject of the complaint. A good example of a formal procedure can be found in the Royal College of Midwives document *In Place of Fear*, or the MSF document *Bullying at Work: Confronting the Problem*, available from the MSF Despatch Department (33-37 Moreland Street, London, EC1V 8BB) at a cost of £10.00. Other policies worth consulting are the Consumers Association Antiharassment Policy and also those produced by the Police and Probation Services.

The Consumers Association uses the following definition:

> *Harassment is behaviour which is unwanted, unreciprocated and offensive to another.*

This is their formal procedure:

The Consumers Association Antiharassment Policy

A *You should register a formal complaint against the alleged harasser. Your complaint should be put in writing to your personnel officer, outlining the nature of the complaint. Your counsellor or staff representative will help you to do this if you wish, but you have the right to initiate a formal complaint without reference to a counsellor first. If your chosen counsellor is also your personnel officer, you may register the formal complaint to the personnel manager, to ensure fairness. In cases involving a senior member of staff the personnel officer's place may be taken by the personnel manager or director of human resources. Throughout the formal process your name and the name of the alleged harasser will not be divulged other than to those who are necessary to the investigation.*

B *The formal complaint will be treated as a disciplinary issue and will be investigated following CA's disciplinary procedure.*

C *A timetable will be set down for the investigation.*

D *There will be an independent investigation carried out by the personnel officer involved in the complaint, to establish the full details of what has happened. You will be interviewed, as will the alleged harasser. Separate interviews will be conducted. Your counsellor or representative will provide help and support during this process if you wish.*

E *The investigation will be thorough, impartial and objective. It will be carried out with sensitivity and with due respect for the rights of both the complainant and the alleged harasser.*

The complainant and the alleged harasser have the right to be accompanied at all interviews. The alleged harasser will be given full details of the nature of the complaint and will be given the opportunity to respond. They will also have access to a counsellor. The investigatory meeting will be held separately and will not be confrontational. Every effort will be made to ensure that the meeting is conducted sensitively.

Strict confidentiality will be maintained throughout the investigation into the allegation. Where it is necessary to interview witnesses, the importance of confidentiality will be emphasised. It will be explained to the witnesses that any breach of confidence would constitute gross misconduct under CA's disciplinary rules and would itself be subject to disciplinary action.

At the completion of the investigation a short report will be prepared summarising the details of the complaint, the results of the investigation and the conclusion. A copy will be sent to both the complainant and the alleged harasser.

If the investigation indicates that harassment has taken place, the harasser will be subject to a disciplinary interview. Depending on the circumstances and the seriousness of the complaint an appropriate penalty will be applied.

If you feel you have been unfairly treated during this procedure you have the right to lodge a grievance using CA's grievance procedure, the last stage of which is an appeal to the director. Ultimately you can take your complaint to an Industrial Tribunal.

Many people who are being bullied do not initiate a complaint, whether formal or informal, because they feel embarrassed, worried that they will not be taken seriously, afraid of further bullying or worried that the perpetrator will 'get into trouble'. Statements to reassure the workforce must be included in the policy and services offered confidentially to ensure that the policy is understood.

Dissemination of information

Any policy is only useful and effective if it is known and understood by the people it is designed to help. Prior to implementation a training or awareness programme should be made available to all members of staff and attendance should be compulsory. This obviously has time and cost implications for a large organisation. Training and information should be included in induction programmes for all new staff. It must be stressed to all staff that this policy covers all staff and that no one is exempt.

The initial financial input may be a factor that prevents large organisations from implementing an effective training programme. It is money well spent when weighed against the increasingly large payouts to victims who claim harassment that are now being reported. It also demonstrates to a tribunal or a court that the employer has attempted to address the problem of bullying within the organisation and has set up internal procedures to help both the victim and the perpetrator. If the victim does not use these pathways then the damages may well be reduced or the claim rejected. Putting money and time into a programme of such training may also increase harmony within the workplace and improve the retention and recruitment of staff. The benefits are always going to outweigh the initial input from the employer!

Any such training programme should be made compulsory for all staff and should be updated on a regular basis. It should be led by a respected training officer, or by an outside agency such as The Industrial Society and should include:

- Initial confirmation that the subjects discussed at the training event will not be recorded or used against any member in the future. A 'safe' environment that encourages disclosures and sharing of experiences should be the aim.

- A discussion on what is meant by bullying and the effects that bullying may have on the individual, whether they are the 'bully', the 'victim' or the 'observer'.

- A discussion on the effects of bullying on the organisation, especially on morale, recruitment and finances if big payouts need to be made.

- Opportunities should be made for the attendees to explore the culture and value systems of the organisation that may have given rise to and perpetuated bullying.

- The policy should be available to every member and it should be 'sold' to them with an emphasis on confidentiality, standard procedures and advice to those who feel that they are being bullied.

- The legal and professional aspects should be included, if only to indicate that this is a nationwide problem, and not a unique occurrence within a particular work environment.

- Training in practical skills such as counselling techniques should be offered to appropriate people.

The policy should be well advertised with up-to-date and informative leaflets to reinforce the training provided and confirm the organisation's commitment. In an organisation in which one of the authors worked, there was a policy in place but few knew about it, even fewer had seen it and because it had not been invoked, the organisation stated that they had no bullying problems! Further information for the employee who feels that she is being bullied can be found in chapter 7.

Genuine shared values

Genuine commitment must be demonstrated by senior management

This has to prove beyond a shadow of a doubt that the organisation is serious in its commitment to erasing bullying and is not just simply paying lip-service to the concept. Antibullying initiatives have to be genuine and applicable to all.

Constant, regular, reinforcement of values

A review of anti-bullying initiatives and reinforcement of management intentions and actions within every appropriate arena or meeting is essential. A 'bully-free zone' is something to be proud of and striven for. Indeed it is essential if the organisation is attempting to create

an environment which is safe, supportive and free from abuse
(UKCC, 1999)

It requires every member of staff to embrace this goal, and to be verbally and formally congratulated when it is achieved. Antiharassment policies must be included in orientation programmes. Staff must be asked at Individual Performance Reviews if they are aware of such policies and arrangements made for updating sessions where appropriate.

Regular monitoring: especially of high-risk, high-stress, 'psychotoxic' working environments

After the initial implementation of any procedures for addressing bullying then things may drift back to the original culture. It is essential to monitor staff attitudes and feelings about bullying on a regular basis and to react accordingly with new initiatives, training or education to ensure that bullying is eradicated constantly. A useful way of monitoring is to ask pertinent questions at exit interviews when staff may no longer be under threat of harassment.

Open-door grievance procedures whereby the aggrieved party is not forced to go through their line manager, who may be the bully

Systems must be in place for individuals or groups to be able to discuss their feelings and/or complaints with an independent and unbiased person or for informal complaints to be made. A specially trained counsellor who may be part of the Human Resource team or Occupational Health team should be available to undertake this important role. A policy that encourages informal complaints can often prevent bullying from causing serious problems.

Know the telltale signs to look for

Systems for monitoring sickness/absence combined with awareness of underlying reasons for patterns of absence can provide an early indication that all is not well. Although work gossip should not be encouraged, sometimes it can give the astute manager hints about bullying. Perhaps an apparently happy and cohesive work group constantly ignores one member of staff. This may represent group harassment of the individual, or that the individual may be the bully. Take seriously informal verbal complaints, even when put forward in a half-joking manner. Give the accuser an opportunity to apply the organisation's policy (if present), and remind the accuser that such complaints can cause problems or be thought of as harassment of the alleged bully by the complainant.

Whilst not wanting to encourage a 'big brother' state within an organisation, the informal support given to and by work colleagues can sometimes mask the true situation from the management. Workers develop a state of acceptance of the situation and believe that there is nothing that anyone can do to improve it because 'it's always been the same'.

Whistle blowers

All NHS Chief Executives would like their organisations to be thought of, by the general public and by their employees, as friendly, supportive and great places to work. The reality, as demonstrated by the research, is often quite different. The public face covers up the unhappiness felt by many who become caught up in the general ethos of the organisation. There is a great reluctance to admit that all is not well in their own particular Garden of Eden. This aggravates the distress of individuals or groups who are made to feel even more out of step with their colleagues. Whether the style of management is one of fear or bonhomie this reluctance to encourage individual complaints and support them to an acceptable outcome is common. The pressure put on employees, or in some cases managers, to fit in with the perceived image of the organisation is a very strong deterrent to complaints. Some large organisations ask employees to sign a contract forbidding them to talk about the organisation outside of their employment. In the NHS there is often an unspoken code for employees not to speak to the media about their place of work in particular or about the NHS in general.

Breaking this code of silence is known as 'whistle blowing' and the most famous recent case was Charge Nurse Graham Pink's attempts to improve standards for the patients in his care by, in desperation, going to the press. This resulted in a much publicised case for unfair dismissal and a costly court case. Graham Pink himself gained a certain notoriety, became one of the best known nurses and was elected to serve as nurse representative on the United Kingdom Central Council in 1993. Later that year the NHS Management Executive issued its 'Guidelines for Staff on Relations with the Public and the Media', designed to make 'whistle blowing' easier.

However, staff are still being disciplined or sacked for making public unacceptable standards of care at work or unjust treatment of staff. Without the right to speak out, some NHS managers and union officials are expressing concerns about deteriorating standards of care in a climate of secrecy. If the threat of action against employees speaking to the media is felt to be real, then there is enormous pressure on a vulnerable employee to 'put up and shut up' when the organisation is treating him/her unfairly.

The RCN document *Whistle blow* (1993) details RCN concerns over the growing use of 'gagging' clauses in employment contracts. These are illustrated as follows:

> *In the course of your normal work with the Trust you will come into the possession of confidential information concerning the Trust and its staff. Such information must always be treated as strictly confidential and, further, must not be divulged to any individual or organisation, including the press, without prior written approval of the Chief Executive or his nominated deputy*

and:

> *Disciplinary action will be taken against any employee who contravenes this regulation.*

These clauses can act in opposition to the UKCC *Code of Professional Conduct* (1992), clauses 1, 2,10 and 11 which state that every nurse, midwife and Health Visitor is accountable for his/her practice and shall:

1 *Act always in such a way as to promote and safeguard the interests and wellbeing of patients/clients.*

2 *Ensure that no action or omission on your part or within your sphere of responsibility is detrimental to the interests, condition or safety of patients/clients.*

It is clear that patient/client care and wellbeing should be paramount when acting as a nurse or midwife. They epitomise the whole reason for the caring professions and the business of healthcare.

10 *Protect all confidential information concerning patients/clients obtained in the course of professional practice and make disclosures only with consent, where*

> *required by the order of the court or where you can justify
> disclosure in the wider public interest.*

11 *Report to an appropriate person or authority, having regard
to the physical, psychological and social effects on
patients/clients, any circumstances in the environment of
care which could jeopardise standards of care.*

Some bullying or harassment of staff by NHS managers can affect the standard of care for vulnerable clients and where all other avenues have been explored these gagging clauses can prevent nurses and midwives from caring for clients to the highest possible standards. Nurses who wrote to the RCN Whistle Blow campaign, sometimes anonymously, used it as a safety valve and there is reason to believe that those being bullied also need this type of support.

> *I am so ashamed that the professional care for whatever reason
> has sunk so low. I just had to get it off my chest.*

> *I do not know what you or anyone else can do, but thank you
> for allowing me to tell someone in safety*

> *I know that writing anonymously doesn't help... but telling
> someone does.*

This campaign also uncovered the fear that many healthcare professionals felt at work. These quotes show how this very real fear affects the individual, the care they give and the organisation that they work for.

> *Anyone who attempts to rectify the situation by approaching
> management is labelled a troublemaker.*

> *We are well represented by our Sister, but we are subject to
> bullying tactics by management.*

> *I have not submitted my name for fear of discrimination.*

> *Two colleagues wrote official letters outlining their very deep
> concerns about [cuts in nursing staff numbers]. Neither received a
> reply for two weeks, but now they have both been informed that
> they are being moved from their wards... Personally I find it all
> rather suspicious that the two who complained are being moved.*

One of the underlying problems that the Whistle Blow campaign revealed was that bullying within the NHS was widespread and almost accepted by the institutions providing healthcare. We have also heard repeatedly that professionals are working within an environment of fear:

> *Morale is low… and staff are frightened and intimidated by a defensive, ingrained management style.*

> *Management are only interested in budgets, not patient care or staff welfare.*

These quotes from the RCN Whistle Blow campaign echoed those of the midwives in our study and the RCM (1996) report. They are not unusual, are heard throughout the UK and are spoken by all grades of staff. It is now clear that bullying, although at the time not recognised as such, has been happening for a long time and we must acknowledge the part that MSF, the RCN and the RCM have played in highlighting the problem.

Some enlightened professional bodies, trade unions and NHS Trusts are now running courses to enable people to use the media well. This should help to encourage an atmosphere of trust between the organisation and the media and remove the threat to the individual who is asked to comment or feels that there is a public interest dimension to information giving. Whilst this is not the norm, it illustrates how powerful organisations can be when they feel threatened and how the individual remains isolated and prevented from seeking assistance and support, even from the organisations and legal systems that are set up to help.

It might be thought that, after the publicity of the RCN campaign, matters would improve, but take heed from this letter, quoted as it appeared in the *Nursing Times*:

> *Take my advice: Speaking out can ruin your life*

> *To any nurse contemplating a grievance procedure, my advice is: stay gagged.*

> *When completing untoward incident forms (which policy dictates) I was told many times that being assaulted was a 'hazard of the job'.*

> *When I reported that patients with dementia in the elderly medical/rehabilitation unit where I worked were indecently and physically assaulting other patients, I was victimised by a senior colleague.*

When I was assaulted by a patient she ignored it. I was in pain and she did nothing to assist. The UKCC said there were no grounds for an inquiry.

I was accused of retaliating against the patient. Management backed my colleague. The tribunal chair accepted untrue and unsigned statements prepared by management and decided I was guilty of misconduct. The union representative was complacent, to say the least.

There is no redress. My 30 years' exemplary service, dedication. concern for patients and staff counted for nothing. Hospital policies and the Patient's Charter put nurses in a no-win situation. Violence and bullying can destroy nurses. I am living proof.

(Name and address supplied)

(Source: *Nursing Times*, Volume 95, No. 19, May 12 1999.)

This situation should now be addressed by the Public Interest Disclosure Act, which was passed in July 1999. The Act gives greater legal protection to employees who blow the whistle on malpractice or wrongdoing in the workplace. It is an extension of the government's moves against gagging\ clauses in employment contracts.

Both employers and unions seem to want to draft internal guidelines to allow staff to be able to 'blow the whistle' in safety. Malpractice or failing to meet agreed standards can be a very costly business for NHS Trusts and any system that raises concerns early is to be recommended. More information on this Act can be obtained from trade unions, professional bodies or from Public Concern at Work, Suite 306, 16 Baldwin Gardens, LONDON EC1N 7RY. E-mail: whistle@pcaw.demon.co.uk. Telephone 0171 404 6609.

Individuals or groups that feel they are being bullied are already in a vulnerable state as their confidence is undermined, their self image diminished and their belief in others damaged. This can cause long and short term effects on their physical, emotional and mental health.

Interventions to reduce stress may target the employee (stress management training), or the environment (stress reduction strategies). Stress management strategies are not common and are rarely provided by employers. Some employees have tried to address stress themselves within groups or teams but unless there is a supportive lead then it often becomes a 'moaning shop' and tends to perpetuate the problems.

The stress that individuals experience can lead to long term health problems, both physical and psychological. Although many ideas have been put forward to manage stress, very few attempts have been made to rectify or manage the causes of the stress.

> *I know there is nothing really wrong with me... I feel so ill at the thought of going to work when X is on duty, but love my job when she is not there. I am ashamed to say that I sometimes ring in sick as I just can't face her... she really does make me feel ill... my head aches, my back hurts and I just feel so tired. I know I should tackle the problem but she could make my life a misery... I think I'll just leave.*

> *I would not recognise that I was under stress, but I knew that my immediate manager was trying to get me moved. I used all the strategies of smiling, relaxation and exercise, tried time management strategies and pushed myself onto all the committees and took on extra work. At the time I was studying for my Master's and had just been through a painful and costly divorce. My father died and I felt I could not even take time off or I would be criticised. At home I was snappy with my family and thoroughly miserable, but I thought I could cope. When I was eventually made redundant the clouds lifted from me and I could feel myself getting back to being the happy, helpful and understanding person I used to be. I dread to think how much further into depression this person could have pushed me.*

Unresolved stress can cause tension headaches and backache, necessitating pain killers or even time off. In some people it affects the alimentary system and aggravates such conditions as Irritable Bowel Syndrome. Some suffer from skin complaints such as eczema or psoriasis. It is well documented that long term stress adversely affects the immune system so that the individual suffers from more colds, sore throats and other opportunistic infections. Stress interferes with sleep patterns, moods and self-image, making the sufferer tired, irritable and unsure of themselves and their decision making. It affects concentration and the ability to care for or about other people or themselves. The person suffering from stress may be tearful, emotionally unstable and lose interest in life. It can lead to a long term depression or to panic attacks.

Post Traumatic Stress Disorder is recognised when people have been involved in unexpected or horrific incidents. Healthcare professionals are expected to cope with these things on a daily basis with no expert help or even recognition. Indeed they are often looked down on if they admit to feelings or emotions about the clients, their role or any other aspect of work. They become labelled as 'sensitive' and may then invite attention from a bullying personality who homes in on anyone who is 'different' or vulnerable.

The effects that these problems have on the workforce, and hence on care provision, should be taken seriously by employers but rarely are. It must be emphasised that stress goes across all levels from the Chief Executive to sessional staff. Bullying and harassment also cross all strata of NHS personnel and it is no coincidence that both of these are unrecognised and/or ignored.

Coping strategies can also be detrimental to the individual or those around them. The most commonly used props for stressed individuals are the easily available and legal remedies of alcohol and cigarettes, with caffeine and chocolate coming a close second. NHS personnel who drink to excess to make stress bearable are soon on a downward spiral; excessive smoking and eating disorders also create long term problems. These can lead to further health problems and time off work and have an adverse effect on self image.

Other ways of coping are to withdraw from life and become isolated, so that time away from work is spent alone, which aggravates depression. Some people exercise to excess. Exercise is good in moderation as it produces endorphins as stress busters, but in excess can become addictive and should be treated as any other addiction. Some of these coping strategies may lead to the illegal use of steroids, amphetamines, cannabis and other drugs. Excessive drinking could lead to driving under the influence of drink especially early in the morning as alcohol takes several hours to be metabolised by the liver. Sometimes stress and/or coping with stress can lead to theft, shoplifting, violence, prostitution and all of these affect the ability of the healthcare worker to care for others. The UKCC Professional Conduct Committee frequently hears cases where nurses and midwives have become embroiled in this kind of downward spiral.

What is not investigated is the root of the individual's problems: these may well be traced back to workplace bullying in some cases. This is an area that managers at local level and those who serve national organisations should begin to question. Every investigation into professional conduct should aim to find out the underlying reasons for a nurse/midwife to change from a confident competent employee to one who has made a small or large mistake. The same questions can be asked at pre-leaving or exit interviews, and when there are requests for transfer of place of work or shift patterns. Only when the right questions are asked will answers be found.

> *The man who does not go down to the underlying causes will never get at the heart of evil.* (Henri de Lubac in *Paradoxes*)

Moving the recipient of bullying may make the victim feel better but will not rout out the perpetrator, who may simply feel more confident and choose another victim.

The importance of recognising the effects of bullying is underestimated by NHS employers. Sometimes the effects of ignoring the health of colleagues or unusual behaviours can have far reaching, even fatal, outcomes. The Allitt inquiry report (Department of Health, 1994) noted that there had been concerns about the behaviour of Nurse Allitt, but nothing had been reported in writing and verbal concerns had not been investigated. The report stipulates that no person in whom there is evidence of major personality disorder should be employed in the nursing profession. MacDonald (1996) extends this definition to include all healthcare staff who may have access to patients.

Within this context, all intimidating and bullying behaviour could be regarded as 'untoward' as it is suggestive of cruelty and lack of conscience. Whilst it is not appropriate for practitioners to undertake personality assessment, untoward incidents should be reported as part of the risk management strategy, so that managers and occupational health staff may take steps to prevent a 'serious untoward incident'. Systems should be in place to screen staff both during recruitment and throughout their employment. This is necessary to prevent a tragedy on the scale of the Allitt case, and also to ensure that bullies are not employed in the first place.

Managers have a moral and legal responsibility not to employ staff who may harm the public and/or their colleagues. However, given the difficulties described earlier, managers have few reliable methods of ensuring staff are 'safe'. Barker et al. (1996) argue that it may be impossible to detect midwives and other staff with personality disorders. They suggest that vast numbers of people move 'in and out' of mental distress and that personality screening and fear of losing one's income may encourage employees to hide their distress rather than be honest and seek help. Porteous (1997) suggests that some staff are more vulnerable to stress than others as a result of differences in coping ability. It could therefore be argued that a dual approach to stress-reduction is necessary, targeting both employees and the working environment.

The Allitt report also highlighted the importance of ward staff in reporting upwards any concerns about a member of staff, and the importance of taking these reports seriously. One of the major omissions of the report was a failure to recommend a counselling and support service. The report recommended several areas where improvements could be made and these included:

The use of common sense and reason.

In these days of staff shortages it is sometimes tempting to employ anyone as a 'pair of hands' even though the manager and other workers know that there are problems concerning that individual. In an attempt to avoid being seen as an unpopular place to work with rapid staff turnover, problems are not addressed and the longer the problem continues the harder it is to deal with.

Managers must take steps to know their staff and not to dismiss intuition.

Happy and successful teams or units at work have a respect for each other and make provision for time out on individual or group activities that enable a relaxed and more intimate knowledge of the individual. Some employees provide for this in quiz nights or sporting activities at reduced or subsidised costs to employees and are supportive of new initiatives for fostering a sense of 'belonging' to the unit/team. Intuition that something is wrong should be brought to a safe listener and steps taken to monitor the situation and provide support to the informer and the person causing concern, without the fear of repercussions.

Be aware of concerns of other staff but avoid tittle-tattle.

If gossip is the main means of communication within an organisation then very little will be changed or taken seriously. It is no joke when people are unwilling to leave a group in case they are the next person to be talked about! Structures should be in place for frank and open discussions of potential problems between staff and managers, without fear of victimisation.

Maintain good links and liaison with education staff.

Since the move of midwifery education into Higher Education premises the links between education and clinical staff need to be nurtured carefully. Sometimes education staff will hear from students of concerns about clinical areas, staff attitudes or competence. The way in which they deal with these concerns can support or hamper good relations. They may simply listen and then dismiss the concern without recording it or referring it to the manager. They may barge into the clinical area with guns blazing and undermine the clinical staff with unproven criticisms from the student, destroying the trust and mutual respect between education and clinical staff. They may record the complaint, and discuss it confidentially with the manager or the person being complained about or take it through a system if one is in place. This latter option relies on good relations already existing between the clinical and education departments.

Provide systems for staff who have concerns.

Policies to support staff, that are known and well publicised, are essential but will only work if there is an atmosphere of trust and confidence. Setting up systems may need new approaches, or even new managers if mistrust is a long seated problem.

Develop mental health policies: it is thought that 30-40% of problems in work are due to mental health problems.

Involvement of occupational health and personnel departments is important, to identify and support those staff who may have problems in this area. It may be necessary to move staff to provide more support or supervision.

> *It is hoped that recent initiatives by the UKCC concerning clinical supervision could help in raising concerns and in supporting nursing and midwifery staff.*

Whilst not the primary aim of clinical supervision, the opportunity to discuss successes and problems at work within a supportive and non-managerial forum could be one way to provide a dedicated listener who can advise, liaise and advocate where problems exist. Where clinical supervision has been successfully implemented staff report positively that their concerns can be heard in a non-judgmental and safe environment which reduces individual and group stress.

Organisational reputation

Organisations which are known to be harsh, uncaring and unhealthy places to work will develop bad reputations which will make recruitment more difficult. Once an organisation has such a reputation it takes major top-down initiatives to address the situation through massive overhaul of the organisational philosophy and culture. This has been illustrated recently in the aftermath to the Stephen Lawrence inquiry: the Chief Constable's resignation was called for because the public had lost confidence in his ability to eradicate the racism inherent throughout the Metropolitan Police Force. This illustrates how important leadership is in organisational change.

Managing change

In the RCM (1996) survey 'change' was cited as a factor which prompted bullying. This included change 'in patterns of care', 'of job', 'of manager', 'to trust status' and 'of supervisor'. If Storr's (1970) assertion that increased competition inevitably leads to increased aggression is correct, the reported increase in bullying with the introduction of NHS Trusts could have been predicted, since the purpose of NHS Trusts was solely to increase competition. In view of the dangers of mental distress, and the increased likelihood of workplace bullying, we suggest that employers should give this subject serious consideration when implementing change or when deciding if change is really necessary.

> *When it is not necessary to change, it is necessary not to change*
> (Lucas Cary, Viscount Falkland d.1643)

Abercrombie (1974) claims that the ability to adapt to change can be in conflict with desirable aspects of the personality such as stability, reliability and trustworthiness. A person who changes their opinions, core beliefs and values frequently (for example, to fit in with current trends) risks being rejected by the group. Aggression can result from observer fear (Hebb, 1973). Observer fear, it is suggested, accounts for the sometimes aggressive and violent reaction of apes when a group member appears to behave strangely through sickness, for example.

When one considers Blane's (1986) assertion that professions are particularly

> *stable and very conservative institutions*

within the context of Storr's (1970) theory on heresy, one can see the potential for increased intimidation when change is proposed within any profession. One could argue that there are important psychological arguments against enforced change, which are often underestimated by managers.

Monitoring the situation is vital, but care must be taken to be supportive and not add to the harassment of individuals. An agreed policy with trade union and professional body involvement is essential. Some important points are worth stressing: sickness and absence costs money that could and should go to improve both patient care and staff support. Concerns should be followed up and sensible guidelines which may indicate the existence of a problem would be:

- over 90 days sickness or absence in 2 years or 10 separate absences in one year
- in excess of 24 days off in one year accrued over at least three periods of absence
- persistent periods of uncertified absence

There seem to be three main types of sickness/absence that raise concerns:

- sporadic uncertified absence of up to 3 days
- regular periods of certified absence
- long-term certified absence.

None of these imply that the 'sickness' is not real: as discussed, the effects of stress can lead to real illness. It is the underlying causes that need to be investigated in a supportive manner, not as a warning to the employee to improve her health but as an opportunity to discuss any underlying problems. It may be worth considering who should undertake this role, as it may be the manager who is the perpetrator of the bullying. Sometimes the occupational health department is the right place for this discussion, sometimes it is the personnel or human resources department. Some enlightened employers provide an outside counsellor to provide this essential service. The employee should be given a choice of people to discuss any problems with.

NHS Trusts and employers need a consistent and adequate system to monitor sickness and absence, to encourage the employee to discuss the underlying reasons for their absence and to give support if stress is at the root of their illness. When trust and confidence in the employer and in the system is present then reporting the cause of the stress may be easier. If bullying or harassment is reported then it should be taken seriously as no one reports this lightly.

Employees or employers can make use of the Health and Safety at Work Act 1974, as bullying that creates stress and ill-health for employees can also contravene the employer's responsibility to their employees.

> *Things do not get better by being left alone. Unless they are adjusted, they explode with a shattering detonation.* (Sir Winston Churchill)

The development of anti-harassment policies is always in danger of being an academic exercise, with the resultant documents being useful for management to quote from. To make create a workable document that is useful to employees takes commitment, time, effort, a respected and persuasive management team and financial support, all of which are in very short supply within the NHS.

Where anti-harassment policies do work, they allow for a safe arena for complaints to be made informally, for the perpetrator and the victim to meet without fear of repercussions, and for a third party to listen, validate their experiences and suggest solutions for progressing the situation whereby both parties feel positive.

The outcome of such interventions should be to allow both parties to feel that they have been allowed to voice their grievances within a neutral and supportive environment. They will feel satisfied that they have not only been heard but have been listened to with respect. Solutions will be reached which may need compromise by each party and also by the organisation.

These strategies do not come cheap, but a caring and forward looking employer knows that this cost is small when compared to the costs that can be incurred with an unhappy workforce. High levels of sickness, absence and mistakes in the NHS can have crippling financial implications and increase recruitment costs where there is poor retention of staff.

Organisations depend on many factors for their success but one of the most important must be reputation. When NHS Trust staff begin to grumble outside the workplace then this delicate reputation can take a battering and the effects can include an increase in staff turnover, a decrease in client numbers, complaints from clients and even the endangerment of the Chief Executive's post. One would think that the time and effort needed to eradicate harassment would be a small price to pay for preserving or improving the reputation of an organisation.

One of the most respected anti-harassment policies can be seen in action in Glasgow, where every member of staff must attend a study day to explore the implications of the policy and the atmosphere within the trust has been enhanced since its introduction. Another manager in the South of England inherited a maternity unit with a reputation of harassment perpetrated by a few powerful people and an atmosphere of fear pervading the work environment. Although much time (and hence money) was required for the manager to interview every member of the staff individually and in confidence, this was the path taken. Gradually, trust in the senior managers replaced the mistrust that had been present and employees began to speak out in unity against some of the practices they had previously put up with. Perpetrators were given opportunities to reassess their attitudes and motives. Many found that it was their own fear of inadequacy that had forced such antisocial behaviour. Opportunities were given for education, relocation if required and in some instances early retirement. Unity of the workforce with common aims and mutual support increased staff confidence in themselves and in their managers. It took about two years for the benefits to be felt in a more stable and happier workforce.

To make an anti-harassment policy work the following points must be considered, or all that will exist will be a document that remains unread, unpractised and unrespected:

- Support and commitment from the highest level possible. This commitment must include time for the policy to be written, discussed, circulated and enacted. There is obviously a financial implication that must be allowed for.

- The involvement of all levels of the institution or organisation, to ensure ownership of the final policy.

- Education, in the form of time out for courses, policy dissemination and for users to define their own needs.

- A high profile for bullying and its sequelae at all meetings, so that people feel comfortable with the twin concepts of acknowledging its existence and erasing it from the organisation.

- Built in mechanisms to allow for celebrations of success, to give positive feedback to those involved and to redefine goals.

- A change agent who is approachable, well known and committed to erasing bullying, to manage, encourage and publicise anti-harassment practices and issues.

Case study

Mrs Johnson, a new manager, was dismayed at the negative atmosphere and fear that could be felt within the organisation she had joined. There was no socialising between groups, rank was pulled at every opportunity and staff sickness and turnover was very high. The hospital had been threatened with closure several years before and investment into the fabric of the buildings and equipment was far from adequate. The morale within all departments was at rock bottom and staff insecurities added to the problems.

Mrs Johnson spent her first month observing interactions between the managers and their staff. She raised problem areas within trust meetings and demanded extra funds to improve working conditions. However, these cosmetic attempts did nothing to improve staff morale.

She then began to invite stewards of the main unions and professional organisations for confidential interview. The unions were not strong within the trust and the stewards felt disinterested as their members did not attend meetings and had given up raising complaints because 'nothing would ever change'.

Applications for further education courses appeared to be non-existent and, after looking into this with the clerical staff, Mrs Johnson discovered that all applications went through a manager who systematically refused them all claiming that there was no money, no replacement staff and that they wouldn't be any use! This had gone on for so long that staff had given up asking for study leave. She then overheard a manager verbally harassing a domestic assistant, calling her 'a lazy cow', and finishing with

all you want to do is to come in and collect your money and none of you ever do any work.

Mrs Johnson arranged to see this manager with the personnel officer. At this meeting she was told that

all the managers speak like that because it is the only way to get staff to work.

She also heard the manager's opinions on second level nurses, care assistants, porters, hospital food, and on the patients, who according to the manager, simply used the hospital when they needed a rest and half of them had nothing wrong with them. After this tirade, which did not appear to be an isolated incident, Mrs Johnson sat for a long time and tried to work out a strategy for turning around this culture of bullying.

A quote from Sir John Moores of the Littlewoods organisation sums up this philosophy. At the time he was talking about equal opportunities, but the ethos applies equally to any anti-bullying policy.

It is not simply about improving the lot of certain groups labelled as 'disadvantaged' but it is actually about having a human resource strategy that both meets the needs of the community and allows [all concerned] to develop their full potential unimpaired by unjustifiable and outmoded systems

He recognised the value and truth of the much quoted statement made by John F Kennedy in 1961:

There are risks and costs to a programme of action. But they are far less than the long range risks and costs of comfortable inaction.

The Industrial Society, in the *Liverpool Echo* (April 26 1999), states:

Staff who are bullied at work could cost their employers up to £200,000 in sick leave, redundancy and pension and other costs.

There are also the effects of worker wastage, retraining, recruitment and retention of staff to consider alongside these costs, not to mention the effect on patient care, which should be the prime consideration of healthcare providers.

Chapter 7

Learning the lessons
The NHS as a developing organisation

Bullying is bad for business

Adams, 1992

Bullying is not only bad for business, it reflects bad management. Effective care and safe working practices can be compromised if managers or staff are suffering stress-related illnesses as a result of being bullied. The high cost of staff turnover and the recruitment and retention problems that can ensue are a burden borne by the organisation that fails to take harassment seriously.

Sickness payments and replacement of staff by agency workers lead to a breakdown in continuity of care and of the good relationships that are enhanced by team working. To this financial burden must now be added the very real possibility of compensation payments to staff who invoke legal redress from an organisation that failed to listen to and act on their complaints.

Persistent harassment of colleagues and/or subordinates is a criminal offence and may contribute to an unsafe environment for workers. If employees or managers suspect colleagues of intimidating or aggressive behaviour within the NHS they, in exercising professional accountability, have a duty to report situations which may endanger patients or colleagues. This could mean defining intimidating behaviour as an 'untoward incident' so that managers can take appropriate action to ensure staff are screened for major personality disorders in accordance with the Allitt inquiry recommendations (Department of Health, 1994). Managers must acknowledge their limitations in personality assessment and request assistance from occupational health departments, staff counsellors and outside agencies.

Organisations should develop an awareness of bullying and managers must take steps to address both the potential and existing problems that it can cause. There must be an assessment of the understanding that staff have of the meaning and effect of bullying, and a method of investigating the extent to which employees feel that they (or their colleagues) are being bullied. Management must be seen to listen to and to take seriously the complaints or comments asked for. Questions should be asked about bullying as a matter of course at exit or transfer interviews, at annual performance reviews and during investigations of other matters such as disciplinary investigations. This is the initial stage in addressing the problem.

As Thomas Henry Huxley so rightly stated in his paper *Aphorisms and Reflections*:

> *My experience of the world is that things left to themselves don't get right.*

Once it is acknowledged that there is a 'problem' that the organisation will not tolerate, management systems have to be designed, applied and evaluated, to enable staff and management to trust each other and to work together in turning around the bullying culture of the organisation.

Practical anti-bullying interventions

It is very helpful to have some knowledge of the legislation around bullying, such as the Sex Discrimination Act of 1975, the Race Relations Act of 1976, the Criminal Justice and Public Order Act of 1994, the Disability Discrimination Act of 1995 and the Protection from Harassment Act of 1997. These are linked to the Health and Safety at Work Act which demands that employers put into practice procedures to protect the safety and health, including the emotional health, of their employees. A definition of what is meant by 'unacceptable behaviour' in the workplace should be included in the policies that form part of the contract of employment.

Bullying or harassment should be defined within every organisation, as some work areas may have different levels of tolerance to others. The input from each member of the organisation must be valued, as this ground work will set the tone and influence the faith of staff in management's ability to influence change.

The formation of an anti-bullying policy is essential. This should be well publicised and will need the provision of workshops and study days to ensure that all employees and managers are aware of the implications for continuing harassment. It should include not only support for the victim of harassment but also help for the perpetrator in the first instance. Failure to comply with the organisation's agreed policies should result in dismissal or even prosecution.

Assessment

Confidential staff surveys should be used to assess the level and nature of bullying within the organisation.

Action initiatives can then be devised to address the bullying culture and turn it around. These can include awareness, training, education, and staff development initiatives such as coaching and mentoring. Regular monitoring and audit of management processes are essential to measure the effectiveness of initiatives and to ensure continual improvement.

Coaching is an unexplored source for potential development. Mentoring schemes have been used in the past with varying degrees of success in the NHS. The success or failure of such schemes often lies in the commitment of the individuals and whether they were allowed to choose their mentor. A framework for employee support and development should be in place which takes account of an individual's need to exercise choice over what areas they need to develop, and who they have as a coach or mentor.

Individuals with sufficient means are now able 'shop around' and hire themselves an external coach who facilitates their personal and professional development. This could be the way forward for the NHS. In light of the difficulties surrounding bullying, it may be asking too much of internal coaches to address this issue. External, independent coaches can more easily challenge individuals if they do not have to work with them on a daily basis. There may also be more trust in the coaching relationship.

Counselling services should be available, either within or outside the organisation, for the support of victims and perpetrators. Many organisations now contract these services to outside bodies in order to ensure that confidentiality and fairness is observed. Counselling should be paid for by the organisation and time given for the employee to attend this form of support. If this support is in place, it may rarely be used once the bullying culture has been turned around.

Stress management services are similar to counselling services, but they are much more directional in helping people to recognise, and build into their lives, effective strategies for coping with stress. Stress is a part of modern day living. The concerned employer will ensure that employees know that the organisation takes this seriously and supports, in practical terms, methods of reducing stress. These may include ensuring that staff are encouraged to take their meal and coffee breaks, a bone of contention throughout the health services and other areas where overwork, under staffing and great responsibility affects the stress levels of individuals detrimentally. Some respected organisations in the commercial sector provide subsidised hair and beauty salons where such treatments as face and hand massages are provided. One Community NHS Trust provides this service, as well as a gym and showering facilities and has found that it is well used by staff. They are monitoring sickness levels to see if there is a decrease over the next year.

Social events such as quiz nights and other leisure activities have been tried and in some circumstances are well used. One trust that was amalgamating three units entered a large team for a women's five kilometre race, and many happy evenings were spent in preparing for this event. As well are having health and mental health benefits to the individual, these events and arrangements also demonstrate that the organisation cares about the employee. The NHS is proud of 'Putting Patients First', but sometimes it is good to 'Put Staff First'.

Training providers should be aware of the short and long term effects of stress on individual health and run sessions to raise awareness of the problems and discuss coping or 'stress-busting' strategies. This may include some radical rethinking on hours worked, shift patterns, and provision of 'time out' during work without being made to feel guilty. Rewards in the form of payment or time off for extra time and duties performed make the employee feel valued, which in recent years has been an unusual emotion! Some organisations arrange block membership of sports or leisure centres or concert venues at reduced prices or even out of hours to help shift workers take advantage of the offer. This is an under-used concession that pays dividends in helping staff to look after themselves and reduce stress.

Coping with stress has to be a partnership between training providers, employees and management to prevent escalation of problems. Although many may be cynical prior to the introduction of such initiatives, a concerted effort, that shows a serious approach and financial input, into looking after staff has been well proven to attract and keep high-calibre staff and enhance the reputation of the organisation. The knock-on effect on client care can also be measured; a happy and cared for workforce can fulfil their role better than a stressed and disillusioned one.

Involvement of unions/professional organisations can assist an organisation in raising problems, supporting people who are being bullied and defining the employment rights and training needs of the perpetrator. They can add validity to the efforts that the organisation is making to eradicate bullying and can ensure that their members are included in discussions, and are given the opportunity to attend information and education sessions so that their grievances are heard and believed.

Development and training

Training in assertiveness skills, to enable individuals to challenge bullying and to stand up to the bully, should be provided either in house or through an outside agency. It should include all employees and managers in multidisciplinary groups. Assertiveness courses help people to practice putting themselves first, to learn not to be taken for granted or made to feel guilty if they refuse a request and to understand the differences between assertive, aggressive, manipulative and passive behaviours. It is also useful to send the bully on these courses as they can be helped to understand why they behave in such a way, can be shown the effects of this on others and can learn how changing their approach can make their working lives happier.

Assertiveness training is often thought to be just about saying 'no', but a more balanced way of delivering courses stresses the negotiation skills required to enable all parties to reach a decision and agree a way of doing things that they each feel happy about: a win-win situation. It is about listening to the other opinions and not just insisting that your own opinion is heard. At the end of negotiation each party should 'feel OK' (Harris, 1973). Negotiation skills are not often taught or employed within the NHS, but should be considered an essential component of management and staff development programmes, and training providers should include access to these in their portfolio of courses.

There is no such thing as constructive criticism. Criticism destroys, feedback nurtures. (Nash and Roger, 1995)

Management development courses should include sessions on how to recognise, and encourage the elimination of, problem behaviours within the organisation. If internal coaching is selected as the way forward, managers should receive quality training in their own coaching skills and staff development courses should include an awareness of coaching and its aims.

Workshops and focus groups are an ideal way to create a forum for staff and managers to discuss the issues within their particular organisation.

Eliminating bullying completely will need thought, a willingness to acknowledge that bullying exists, the courage to take up the initiatives and the negotiation skills to divert funds and time to eradicating it. The authors do not consider that this is an easy task as the manager sometimes feels that she alone has to turn around the whole culture of an organisation and act ruthlessly to support the statement that bullying will not be tolerated. Since the NHS is a national organisation, and NHS culture is widespread and not confined to isolated units, it must be noted that local initiatives alone are unlikely to achieve permanent widespread change without NHS executive support at national level.

It is also necessary these days to ensure that the education establishments are aware of and support the initiatives and policies of the healthcare provider and work to the same standards. Education staff have the same responsibilities towards their students and the clinical staff who work with them as the managers of the organisation and should be included in the dissemination and implementation of any anti-harassment policy that is in place where students are gaining experience. Antibullying initiatives apply to education managers too!

From reactive to proactive

'Proactive' has been a buzzword for so long that few people stop to consider its actual meaning, let alone ask themselves, how do we get from reactive to proactive in an organisation like the NHS?

The NHS often suffers from the fact that, as an organisation, it lacks a central purpose. Modern organisations have a clear aim or 'mission statement' so that everyone working within the organisation is clear about what they are trying to achieve. Within the NHS, nursing and midwifery staff believe they are there to provide the best quality care available ('Total Quality'), yet managers are told they are to remain within a fixed budget and all too often that budget is reduced. These aims are contradictory: you wouldn't expect to be able to get the finest haute cuisine in Britain's top restaurant for the same price as a 'happy-burger' meal! Yet that is exactly what we are expecting from the NHS: we expect the best yet we don't want to pay for it.

An interesting commentator on this subject is Seedhouse (1995), who describes the 'siege mentality' in the NHS that results from this lack of a clear philosophy. Each hospital, and indeed each department, is competing for resources; they do not view themselves as teams working together with common values towards a common aim.

A clear aim, to give the organisation a sense of purpose, is essential, and this is especially true where resources are scarce. Much stress arises from disagreements on how to allocate scarce resources and competition in acquiring those resources. Such 'fire-fighting' does not allow managers to develop creativity, initiative, and innovating skills.

There is no longer a social consensus that the health services exist for the common good. Whilst Seedhouse (1995) argues that the NHS lacks an overall philosophy, Nettleton (1995) suggests that the health professions, such as midwifery, are self-serving. The authoritarianism of the early midwives, discussed in chapter 2, would be perceived, in the context of contemporary society, as aggressive, intimidating or even criminal!

Making a real difference

There will, undoubtedly, be some staff whose aggression is a sign of a personality disorder. There will be other staff and patients whose aggression is a response to the hostile environment of the hospital, and possibly many more whose aggression results from being unable to cope with stress. Neither a witch-hunt nor burying our heads in the sand will help. What is required is a rational, intelligent risk management strategy to reduce associated factors such as stress and increase support, not only for nurses and midwives, but for all NHS employees and carers.

IPR and attitude testing can show managers where behaviour such as bullying, racism or sexism exists. Coaching can make a real difference in developing these individuals so that they can move forward and be a contributing member of the team once more. We prefer the term coaching to mentoring because of the association with action and movement. Effective coaching demands a move forward or progress towards a goal, otherwise what is the difference between coaching and conversation? Staff with health problems, whose development is temporarily blocked, can be helped through occupational health and may be offered counselling. All staff, where performance issues have been identified, should be offered one of these options proactively as part of the organisation's risk management strategy. Staff with serious personality disorders, displaying potentially harmful behaviour, such as Beverley Allitt, should be suspended pending enquiry and subsequent dismissal. Management systems should allow for staff to report, without fear of recrimination, when a colleague's behaviour is 'untoward'. Stress management training would improve individuals' coping abilities whilst organisation-wide stress reduction strategies could reduce the stress levels within the work environment and target areas where action is needed.

Support for midwives

Midwifery supervision deserves a special mention here because Supervisors of Midwives were implicated both in the RCM report and in the cases reported to us. For the information of non-Midwifery Managers it must be noted that the Supervisor of Midwives is a statutory role and is not to be confused with supervisory management. It has to be said though, that there has been much confusion in this regard in the past, and perhaps a change of title for the statutory supervisory role would be the best way forward to avoid further confusion.

Demilew (1995) argues that midwifery supervision is often practised in a controlling, negative and obstructive way. In contrast, Taylor (1995) offers a model based on those used in counselling, which is positive, supportive and non-judgemental. A move towards the latter might be necessary if midwives are to feel comfortable to discuss their anxieties and explore solutions.

Action checklist for managers

❏ Develop awareness: make sure everyone understands the legislation and is aware of their responsibilities.

❏ Agree on a working definition.

❏ Involve staff-side organisations as early as possible.

❏ Develop trust and effective two-way communication. This includes effective listening.

❏ Formulate an anti-bullying policy.

❏ Carry out a confidential survey of employees at all organisational levels.

❏ Set up bully-free management processes, such as open-door grievance procedures.

❏ Plan and implement continuous employee training, support and development, for both staff and management.

❏ Create an infrastructure to provide this, including coaching and counselling services.

❏ Devise a dual approach to stress-management, tackling the environment as well as individuals.

❏ Carry out regular audit of management processes and anti-bullying initiatives.

What to do if you are being bullied

1. Record what has happened

The most useful advice that anyone can give to someone who is being bullied is to keep a written record of what has happened. This should include the date and time of the incident, who else was present, the circumstances around the incident and exactly what was said or what happened. Your feelings at the time and any action that you took afterwards should also be recorded. Although at first it may seem trivial, the record of several incidences including the same person or people and similar feelings afterwards are essential to prove a case.

A record may look something like this:

> *May 3 1999 around 12.30 in the hospital canteen. Mary J came over to me and told me that I couldn't change my off duty with Sally P. When I asked why, she said because the sooner I learnt to stick to the off duty given the better. When I said that I had requested Saturday off, she told me that if I made a fuss she would see to it that I would never get another Saturday off while she was in charge. This is the way that she speaks to me all the time and I feel as though I just don't want to work here any more.*

> *May 10 1999 4.45pm in the changing room. Mary J came in as I was getting ready to go home and told me that the ward was in a mess and that it was all down to me for never tidying up after myself. I said that I had put everything away that I had used but she insisted that I got back into uniform and went back to the ward to tidy up. No one else was around as they had all got off on time, it was only me who had stayed late. I went back with her but could find nothing wrong, so she said that someone else must have done it for me, again. By the time I got changed again I had missed my train and was late collecting my daughter from her child minder. This made me feel very guilty and angry that I had once more allowed Mary to upset me.*

> *May 15th 1999 3pm in the ward by Mrs Smith's bed. Nurse Sally P was present when Mary J came over and told me that I was the worst nurse she had ever had on the ward and the sooner I moved somewhere else the better. When Sally asked her what I had done she just said, 'she knows' and walked off. I spent the rest of the day and night wondering what I had done wrong. The patient said she got upset because Mary J was always picking on me and said that I should complain. I have asked for a transfer but haven't heard anything.*

Many similar entries would provide excellent evidence and memory-joggers if or when a complaint was made. As is often the case in other areas of nursing and midwifery, contemporaneous and correct records can make the difference between a successful and an unsuccessful outcome.

If a single incident is particularly worrying, you can go to a solicitor and ask to swear an affidavit. This just means that the solicitor records the incident and you swear a legal statement to the solicitor that the events are true to the best of your knowledge and belief. This is then recorded, dated and signed. In the event that a case is brought in future months or years, sworn affidavits hold more weight in court because they indicate that you must have been sufficiently concerned to go to the trouble of making one.

2. Tell someone

It is important that you share your concerns and feelings about what has happened with someone else. This may be a family member, a work colleague or someone whose advice and experience you trust. Very often the person being bullied complains to friends and family so often that people begin to dread being in contact with them. Although this off-loading is an important component of trying to make sense of a terrible situation, it does nothing to 'cure' the situation. A trusted confidante, though, is useful to support you through the process of making a complaint. You may choose to tell your personnel officer or manager but only if you feel confident that they will believe you and that they will help you to do something constructive about it.

Although it may give you a temporary respite from the stress of meeting the bully, it is no good in the long run simply moving you away from the bully. She/he will then pick on someone else, and you will not have been given the opportunity to deal with your feelings about being bullied and grow from them. Some people feel more comfortable talking to their union steward who can offer support and take any complaints further.

3. Decide on a plan of action

This will depend on many things. You may decide to talk to your colleagues and see if they have experienced the same treatment and would support a group complaint. If you are the only one, this will help you to find out who would support you if you took a complaint forward.

Sort out copies of your annual appraisals, education requests, refusals or certificates. Update your personal professional profile and include any cards or letters that you have had from patients/clients or students that support, praise or appreciate your work. Get a copy of your job description and make sure that you are meeting the responsibility criteria it sets down. Write down any areas where you are working above your grade or have asked for experience or education and it has been denied.

Ask your personnel department whether your organisation has a policy on bullying or harassment. If so, request a copy and read it. Remember that these policies are often worded in unfamiliar language so you could ask a personnel manager to explain it and use hypothetical examples to see if your complaint would be covered by it. Keep records of any appointments with your GP or any other therapist and their treatment or advice, along with any health complaints or stress related symptoms, with dates so that these could be cross referenced if required.

You may decide to challenge the bully and make it clear that you will not put up with their behaviour any longer. State that if it continues you know your rights and will take it further. Record this meeting and what the reaction was, with the date. It may be useful to have a witness.

If there is no improvement then the next step is to make a complaint using the harassment policy if there is one in place. Ask your union or professional organisation representative to do this with you.

It is important to be clear about what you want the outcome to be and to stick to your requests, using the 'broken record' technique that is taught at assertiveness classes. Your may want an acknowledgement that bullying has occurred, and you may want an apology. You may want to get the bully transferred or removed from working with you.

In some cases where bullying has had a severe effect on your health, whether physical or psychological, or on your income, then financial compensation may be what you want. Your union or legal representative will advise you on what is possible and what is probable.

Your complaint can in the first instance be made to whoever you feel will believe you and support you to take it forward. Although line management may be recommended you can go straight to the top, or through personnel or occupational health departments if you prefer. It is definitely not recommended to go for any publicity before or during any complaint procedure, as this may jeopardise any legal proceedings in the future.

An informal investigation may happen first, followed by a formal investigation if no agreement is reached. If the organisation fails to believe you or to take action on your behalf, you may be able to take legal action against them to gain compensation for the stress and/or loss of earnings that may have been caused by this.

4. Know your rights, and tell others about them.

Only when the majority of the workforce care enough about bullying will changes to the bullying culture occur.

5. Take steps to rebuild your self-esteem.

Bullies target people they feel are weak and vulnerable. Sometimes the victim begins to act out those attributes; if you have been told that you are always miserable it is difficult to act in a carefree manner. If you are told over and over again that you are hopeless and forgetful, eventually you begin to doubt your own abilities and become forgetful through stress. If the bully says that no one likes you, it is easy to misinterpret off hand remarks from colleagues in a negative way and begin to think that the bully is right.

You need the support of your family, work colleagues, friends and union whilst you are going through a complaints procedure. Many people find that the whole experience makes them stronger and they become more assertive and proactive for others, but others find that their self image has been dented and begin to feel that somehow they deserved the treatment they attracted. The development of this mentality then makes it more likely that the bullying will recur, so reinforcing their opinion. This is more common if childhood experiences have also occurred that have put the individual in the victim role. To break this cycle there may need to be positive interventions such as assertiveness training or counselling. The employer should have facilities for this to be arranged within or outside the organisation to enable the individual to grow stronger from the experience and not to suffer further damage. If these are not offered or available through your workplace then look in your local library, health centre or further education college for courses or counselling that may help you.

Sometimes writing about your experiences in a personal diary helps, especially if you can identify the feelings and emotions that you have felt.

These may link with similar feelings in other areas of helplessness and remembering how you managed them in one set of circumstances may give you some ideas about how to cope now and in the future. The more you talk and think about what has happened in the early stages the better. Feelings that are not acknowledged can fester, creating more stress and unresolved anger which can cause more problems later.

What to do if you feel you may be a bully

It may be that reading this book has triggered minor or major guilt feelings that you may have been a bully. Everyone is probably guilty at some time of verbal abuse of another person, especially when under stress at work or home. Often we are sorry for the things that we have said and feel for the person we have abused. A well-timed apology and acknowledgement that we were wrong usually makes everything all right as that person knows that we have acted out of character and they often kindly make excuses for our behaviour.

This book is not about everyday and acceptable slips in good behaviour but about the systematic and often premeditated verbal or physical abuse or undermining of another. We have touched briefly on racial, age and sexual discrimination and most people understand the seriousness of these. Many psychologists would say that bullies are inadequate or damaged people who need to feel superior to someone and home in on a victim and proceed to humiliate them for sheer pleasure.

In the real world, most bullies do not stop to analyse why they do things, or what effect they are having. They may just believe that they are right to try to 'get rid' of a person that they feel is not pulling their weight in a team or maybe they feel that someone else would do the job better. They may feel threatened by someone who is younger, more experienced, more popular, more qualified or may feel inadequate within their role and unhappy because of circumstances outside work. They may have been bullied in the past and are now determined to 'retaliate first' so that it does not happen again. If you can identify yourself in any of these descriptions then you are now on the way to tackling the bullying problem!

Most bullies do not feel remorse for their behaviour as they think that they are acting in the cause of the common good and would be horrified to find their behaviour being called 'bullying'. If you are confused about this, find out if your organisation runs study sessions on bullying or is setting up an anti-harassment policy and get involved. Bullies are not universally loved as they attempt to save the world from inadequate people, even though their motives for doing so can be supported!

Looking at the cause and effect of behaviour in a safe environment such as counselling or role play is sometimes useful. When you have had a bad day at work take some time to think through who you have spoken to, who has upset you and who you may have upset. Try to define your feelings about each transaction. Look at the interactions that made you feel bad and try to find out why. Think how the other person may have felt. Now look at the interactions that have made you feel good, and consider why this may have been. Think how the other person may have felt. If you think they may have felt upset, frightened or inadequate as a result of their interaction with you, and if this person features frequently in interactions with this outcome, then you may have a problem with bullying.

The aim of caring interpersonal interactions is to end each episode with each participant 'feeling OK' (Harris, 1973) about it. How can you make this happen?

- Do you feel that you are under such stress that you may need help to change your attitude and temper control?

- Do you need to talk to someone about coping with stress?

- Have you identified yourself as being more aggressive than assertive?

- Are you generally unhappy at work or/and home?

If you have answered 'yes' to any of these questions then now is the time to take back control of your life. You may want to start by speaking to your General Practitioner if you have any underlying or long-term health problems: ask if he can recommend a course of action for you to start.

Sometimes health workers neglect their own health and fitness at the expense of caring for their patients and/or family. Consider your lifestyle and make changes that will help you towards fitness. Hiring a personal coach helps you to make real, personal changes.

Find out if there are any classes in your area to help you manage stress, develop assertiveness and control aggressiveness. Sometimes it helps to talk to a counsellor if you feel you have deep rooted problems that you have not addressed. Your employer may be able to arrange this for you if you ask through your occupational health department.

Try reading some of the self-development books that help people to take control of their lives and start the journey to happiness. The aim is to be happy, however you may define that state for you.

Once you have begun some of these steps, you are well on the way towards managing bullying within yourself and this will have an immediate effect on your interactions with colleagues. Of course, it may take them longer to accept the changes that you are making internally, but don't give up, they will eventually respond and give you the opportunity to develop good relationships.

What to do if you are accused of being a bully

If someone has named you in a complaint, do not panic and start to go after the person you think has complained, in an attempt to force them to withdraw their complaint. This would only add to the evidence and support the complaint.

It is important to remain as calm as possible and get some support as you will need someone to talk to while the process takes place. This may be your line manager, a personnel officer or your steward from your union or professional organisation. It is not usual for details of the complaint or the complainant to be given to you when you are first informed but it is useful if you look back at any interactions with staff to see if you could have been misinterpreted. Sometimes a bully will make a complaint if they think that they are about to be the subject of a complaint. Spend some time collecting evidence to support your standards of care and loyalty to the organisation such as letters or cards of thanks from patients, relatives or students, and make sure that your professional profile is up to date.

A meeting will be arranged between the managers, personnel and you and your support person. Try to stay calm and listen to the complaints.

If these are untrue then say so. If the complaints are a misinterpretation of what you intended to convey then listen carefully to the allegations, carefully making any notes you might need, then leave the room to gather your thoughts before you answer them. Make an appointment to return with your representative, then explain the circumstances and state that you are sorry that your words were misinterpreted and you have caused someone to be upset.

The investigating panel will try to decide on a course of action to help both you and the complainer to feel that they have been listened to and positive action is the outcome.

If you feel that there are areas where you need help such as extra staff over busy times, a different form of off duty allocation or any other positive suggestions for improvement then this is an opportunity to put forward your requests, to avoid such explosive incidents occurring in future. If you feel that you need personal help in the form of counselling, stress management or even time off to deal with other problems that are impinging on work then this is the time to ask for them. Remember that the panel want to help to avoid any costly payout to the complainer!

You may want to ask for a transfer or early retirement, but only do this if you really want to and do not just use it as an opportunity to run away from the problem. Finally, use the services of your union or professional organisation. That is why you have paid your subscription and they are the experts in advising and supporting their members in such upsetting incidents.

Conclusion

Bullying behaviour is complex, difficult to define and equally difficult to observe or study. It can be intentional or unintentional. It may be subjective or it may form part of a complex network of interactions between individuals within a group. Certainly in midwifery, a strict, ruthless approach has been encouraged in the past and possibly perpetuated as part of the professional subculture. In modern society this could be perceived at least as insensitivity, at most as intimidating behaviour. The origins of intimidating behaviour are multifactorial, being influenced by both intrinsic and extrinsic factors.

Workplace bullying is destructive wherever it occurs, but there are serious implications for the NHS. Strategies must be adopted to prevent another Allitt case, yet workplace eugenics which exclude the sick and disabled from the workplace are illegal and immoral. Nurses and midwives have a legal responsibility to protect the public and their colleagues. However, nursing and Midwifery Managers are sometimes those responsible for bullying (RCM, 1996). It must not be assumed that managers are exempt from personality disorders. Preventative strategies must therefore be applied equally to all NHS employees, including senior management.

Increased competition within the NHS has contributed to increased bullying. Hopefully the dismantling of the internal market will redress the balance. Risk management could be the most important management intervention pertinent to this issue. Ongoing systems of staff support and development, provided either internally or by an outside agency, which balance coaching and counselling, are essential. In struggling to achieve targets with finite resources NHS managers should at least ensure that harm is not done. The adoption of a single NHS philosophy could focus managers on the ultimate goal.

The professional subculture which enabled authoritarianism to thrive needs to be addressed throughout the professions, but especially in the areas of education and clinical supervision where a supportive environment must be created to facilitate personal and professional development. Due to the deeply entrenched nature of bullying within the NHS and educational institutions it may be necessary for NHS Trusts that are serious about addressing this issue to engage external consultants. In view of the potential harm that can result, it is essential that nursing and midwifery staff are able to recognise when their behaviour could be perceived as aggressive, intimidating or bullying.

Behaviour which at the beginning of the 20th century was considered desirable and necessary has become, at the beginning of the 21st century, criminal. According to Storr (1970):

> *...the heresy of one generation may well become the orthodoxy of the next.*

It appears that the reverse is also true. Even if every recommendation in this book were implemented tomorrow it would be out of date in ten years time. The true way forward is for the NHS to have a clear vision, to strive united towards that vision and to fully embrace a culture of change as a developing organisation. Lifelong learning applies to organisations as well as to the individuals within, and ongoing support structures which facilitate personal, professional and organisational development are vital, whether provided internally or externally.

Further reading

Adult Bullying: Perpetrators and victims.
Randall P. London: Routledge, 1997.

Bullying at Work: How to confront and overcome it.
Adams A. London: Virago, 1992.

Games People Play.
Berne E. New York: Grove Press, 1964.

Grooming, Gossip, and the Evolution of Language.
Dunbar R. London: Faber & Faber, 1996.

NLP at Work.
Knight S. London: Nicholas Brealey, 1995.

The Nurture Assumption.
Harris JR. London: Bloomsbury Publishing, 1999.

Contacts and resources

CONSULTANTS

Ruth Hadikin Associates:
Coaching, development and training consultancy.
Contact Ruth Hadikin: 01704 896039.
E-mail RHAssocs@aol.com.
Http://www.ruthhadikin.com

Healthfirst Consultants:
Stress management, employee counselling,
expert witness for midwifery, stress, PTSD.
Contact Muriel O'Driscoll: 0151 928 0596.
E-mail muriel@healthfirstconsultants.co.uk.
Http://www.healthfirstconsultants.co.uk

HELPLINES

Bullying Helpline
0181 885 1677

Imperative
01983 856379 (Monday to Friday 8.00-10.00pm)

Workplace Bullying Hotline
01235 834548

Bully Alert UK
01227 277993 for NHS and voluntary sector workers.

Peach Stop the Bullying Helpline
01582 612734 (Mon, Wed and Thurs 7.30-9.30pm).

The Department of Health
Information Line number is 0800 555 777.
website is http://www.doh.gov.uk

LITERATURE AND RESOURCES

Bullying at Work: Confronting the problem
is available from the MSF Despatch Department,
33-37 Moreland Street, London, EC1V 8BB at a cost of £10.

In Place of Fear:
Recognising and confronting the problem of bullying in midwifery
Available from The Royal College of Midwives,
15 Mansfield Street, London W1M 0BE £10.

The I-A-B Developmental Tool
Available from Ruth Hadikin Associates, details as above.

We Don't Have To Take This
a resource pack containing information on the government's NHS zero
tolerance zone initiative.
Available free from the NHS Responseline on 0541 555455.

The Provision of Counselling Services for Staff in the NHS:
Moving staff support up the agenda
a document outlining the NHS Executive guidance on staff
counselling,
Will be available from the NHS Responseline on 0541 555455,
sometime during 2000 though the exact date was not available at the
time of going to press.

Copies of the report by The Institute of Work Psychology at the
University of Sheffield and the Psychological Therapies Research
Centre at the University of Leeds by Borrill CS et al. can be obtained
from Nicky Wheeler on 0114 222 3266 for a small charge.

More information on *The Public Interest Disclosure* Act can be
obtained from trade unions, professional bodies or from Public
Concern at Work, Suite 306, 16 Baldwin Gardens, London EC1N
7RY. E-mail: whistle@pcaw.demon.co.uk. Telephone 0171 404 6609.

The National Association for Staff Support contact address is
NASS, 9 Caradon Close, Woking, Surrey, GU21 3DU
Telephone 01483 771 599.

References

Abercrombie MLJ. (1974) *The Anatomy of Judgement.* Middlesex: Penguin.

Adair J. (1987) *Effective Teambuilding.* (2nd edn.) London: Pan books.

Adams A. (1992) *Bullying at Work: How to confront and overcome it.* London: Virago.

Adorno TW, Frenkel-Brunswick E, Levinson D and Sanford N. (1950) *The Authoritarian Personality.* New York: Harper.

Allcock L. (1995) *Psychology in Practice.* London: Southbank University.

Allen RE. (Ed) (1990) *The Concise Oxford Dictionary of Current English.* (8th edn.) Oxford: Clarendon.

Asch SE. (1946) Forming Impressions of Personality. *Journal of Abnormal and Social Psychology* 41: 258-90.

Bakal DA. (1979) *Psychology and Medicine: Psychobiological dimensions of health and sickness.* London: Tavistock.

Bakker RHC, Groenewegen PP, Jabaaij L, Meijer W, Sixma H, de Veer A. (1996) 'Burnout' among Dutch midwives. *Midwifery* 12(4), 174-81.

Bandura A. (1977) *Social Learning Theory.* Englewood Cliffs, NJ: Prentice-Hall.

Barker P, Reynolds B, Whitehill I, Novak V. (1996) Working with mental distress. *Nursing Times* 92(2), 25-7.

Berne E. (1964) *Games People Play.* New York: Grove Press.

Blane D. (1986) Health Professions. In: Patrick DL, Scambler G. (Eds.) *Sociology as applied to medicine.* Eastbourne: Baillière Tindall.

Borrill CS. (1998) *Stress Among Staff in NHS Trusts* (unpublished research report).The Institute of Work Psychology: University of Sheffield and The Psychological Therapies Research Centre: University of Leeds.

Calnan M. (1987) *Health and Illness: The lay perspective.* London: Tavistock. Cited by: Nettleton S. (1995) *The Sociology of Health and Illness.* Cambridge: Polity.

Child D. (1986) *Psychology and the Teacher.* London: Cassell Education.

Clark E, Keeble S.(1995) *Introduction to Psychological Knowledge.* London: Southbank University.

Daley M, Wilson M. (1988) *Homicide.* New York: Aldine.

Demilew J. (1995) Examples of Good Supervision. In: Association of Radical Midwives (Eds) *Super-Vision: Consensus conference proceedings.* Manchester: Books for Midwives Press.

Department of Health. (1994) *The Allitt Inquiry: Report of the independent inquiry relating to the deaths and injuries on the children's ward at Grantham and Kesteven general hospital during the period February to April 1991.* London: HMSO.

Department of Health. (1993) *Changing Childbirth Part 1: Report of the Expert Maternity Group.* London: HMSO.

Dimond B. (1999) Stress and the Midwife. *British Journal of Midwifery* 7(10), 649.

Dunbar R. (1996) *Grooming, Gossip, and the Evolution of Language.* London: Faber & Faber.

Eysenck HJ. (1965) *The Structure of Human Personality.* London: Methuen & Co. Ltd.

Field T. (1996) *Bully in Sight: How to predict, resist, challenge and combat workplace bullying.* Oxford: Success Unlimited.

Flinn MW. (1977) *An Economic and Social History of Britain since 1700.* London: Macmillan.

Flint C. (1993) *Midwifery: Teams and caseloads.* Oxford: Butterworth Heinemann Ltd.

Griffiths D. (1981) *Psychology and Medicine.* London: Macmillan.

Hadikin R, O'Driscoll M.(1997) Interpersonal Skills. In: Henderson C, Jones K. (Eds) *Essential Midwifery.* London: Mosby.

Hadikin R. (1998) The impact of the recommendations of *Changing Childbirth* on Community Midwifery practice. *MIDIRS Midwifery Digest* 8(1), 12-4.

Hadikin R. (1997) The state of midwives' pay. *MIDIRS Midwifery Digest* 7(3), 280-3.

Halsbury's Statutes (1997) *Current Statutes Service* (Issue 76). London: Reed Elsevier.

Haralambos M. (1987) *Sociology: A new approach.* Ormskirk: Causeway Press.

Harré R. (1979) *Social Being: A theory for social psychology.* Oxford: Basil Blackwell Ltd.

Harris JR. (1995) Where is the Child's Environment? A group socialization theory of development. *Psychological Review* 102(3), 458-89.

Harris TA. (1973) *I'm OK–You're OK.* New York: Avon.

Hebb DO.(1973) *The Organization of Behavior.* New York: Wiley.

Heider F. (1958) *The Psychology of Interpersonal Relations.* New Jersey: Lawrence Erlbaum.

Hicks C. (1995) Good researcher, poor midwife: An investigation into the impact of central trait descriptions on assumptions of professional competencies. *Midwifery* 11(2), 81-7.

Hunt S, Symonds A. (1995) *The Social Meaning of Midwifery*. Hampshire: Macmillan.

Ingham R, Fielding P. (1985) A review of the nursing literature on attitudes towards old people. *International Journal of Nursing Studies* 22, 171-81.

Jowitt M. (1997) Letters: Editor's note. *Midwifery Matters* 74, 38.

Kline P. (1981) Personality and Individual Assessment. In: Griffiths D. (Ed) *Psychology and Medicine*. London: Macmillan.

Knight S. (1995) *NLP at Work*. London: Nicholas Brealey.

Leap N, Hunter B. (1993) *The Midwife's Tale*. London: Scarlet Press.

Lyons R, Tivey H, Ball C. (1995) *Bullying at work: How to tackle it. A guide for MSF representatives and members*. London: MSF.

MacDonald A. (1996) Responding to the results of the Beverley Allitt inquiry. *Nursing Times* 92(2), 22-5.

May WF. (1975) Code, covenant, contract, philanthropy. *Hastings Centre Report* 5, 29-38.

Morris D. (1989) *Manwatching: A field guide to human behaviour*. London: Grafton.

MSF (1994) *Bullying at work: Confronting the problem*. London: MSF.

Nash P, Roger D. (1995) Get Ahead. *Nursing Times* 91(31), 44-5.

Nettleton S. (1995) *The Sociology of Health and Illness*. Cambridge: Polity.

NHS Executive. (1991) *NHS Research and Development Strategy: Guidance for regions*. London: Department of Health.

Oakland JS. (1993) *Total Quality Management*. Oxford: Butterworth Heinemann.

O'Driscoll M. (1997) Redundancy: The end or the beginning? *MIDIRS Midwifery Digest* 7(4), 422-3.

Porteous M. (1997) *Occupational Psychology*. Hemel Hempstead: Prentice Hall.

Quine L. (1999) Workplace Bullying in NHS Community Trust: Staff questionnaire survey. *British Medical Journal* 318, 228-32.

Randall P. (1997) *Adult Bullying: Perpetrators and victims*. London: Routledge.

Rayner C, Hoel H. (1997) A summary review of literature relating to workplace bullying. *J Comm Appl Soc Psychol.* 7, 181-91.

Rees L. (1997) *The Nazis: A warning from history*. London: BBC Books.

Reich B, Adcock C. (1976) *Values, Attitudes and Behaviour Change*. London: Methuen

Rogers CR. (1989) *On Becoming a Person: A therapist's view of psychotherapy*. London: Constable.

Royal College of Midwives. (1996) *In Place of Fear: Recognising and confronting the problem of bullying in midwifery*. London: RCM.

Sandall J. (1997) Midwives burnout and continuity of care. *British Journal of Midwifery* 5(2), 106-11.

Seaman B. (1995) Where Supervision Goes Wrong. In: Association of Radical Midwives (Eds) *Super-Vision: Consensus conference proceedings*. Manchester: Books for Midwives Press.

Seedhouse D. (1995) *Fortress NHS: A philosophical review of the national health service*. Chichester: Wiley.

Shapiro DA. (1981) Psychopathology. In: Griffiths D. (Ed) *Psychology and Medicine*. London: Macmillan.

Silverman D, Gartrell N, Aronson M, Steer M, Edbril S. (1983) In Search of the Biopsychosocial Perspective: An experiment with students. *American Journal of Psychiatry* 140, 1154-9.

Steinaker NW, Bell MR. (1979) *The Experiential Taxonomy*. New York: The Academic Press.

Storr A. (1970) *Human Aggression*. Middlesex: Penguin.

Tannen D. (1992) *You Just Don't Understand: Women and men in conversation*. London: Virago.

Tannen D. (1998) *The Argument Culture: Changing the way we argue and debate*. London: Virago.

Taylor M. (1995) Psychodynamic Counselling and Therapy. In: Association of Radical Midwives (Eds) *Super-Vision: Consensus conference proceedings*. Manchester: Books for Midwives Press.

The Guardian (1995) News In Brief (editorial). *The Guardian*, July 10, 1995.

United Kingdom Central Council for Nursing, Midwifery, and Health Visiting. (1992) *Code of Professional Conduct for the Nurse, Midwife and Health Visitor*. London: UKCC.

United Kingdom Central Council for Nursing, Midwifery and Health Visiting. (1993) *Midwives Rules*. London: UKCC.

United Kingdom Central Council for Nursing, Midwifery, and Health Visiting. (1999) *Practitioner-Client Relationships and the Prevention of Abuse*. London: UKCC.

Wells C. (1997) Stalking: The criminal law response. *Criminal Law Review* 765, 463-70.

Index

Absenteeism, 9, 21, 83–4, 130,
   142–3
Abuse, 91, 100
Accountability, 112–14
   case studies, 113, 114
Actor-observer bias, 51
Affective aggression, 66
Aggression, 37–9, 44, 58–9,
   65–6
   affective, 66
   definition of, 116–17
   heresy factor, 59–61
   instrumental, 66
   observer fear and, 142
   psychological theories of,
      44–5
   see also Bullying; Harassment
Alcohol intake, 89
Anger, 49
Anti-harassment policy, 124–8,
   143–5, 151
   see also Organisational
   culture change
Assault, 100–1, 113
Assertiveness training, 154
Assessment of bullying, 152–4
Attitudes, 54
Attribution theory, 52–3
   case study, 52–3
   gender difference, 53
   sexual harassment and, 53–4
Authority, 39–40

male-dominated hierarchies,
   40–1

Body language, 69
Bullies:
   personality traits of, 65–6
   procedure for, 163–5
Bullying, 8–11, 166–8
   among midwives, 1–3, 9,
      11–12, 22, 86–91
      case studies, 23–4, 86–7,
         90–1
      Supervisors, 22–3, 25
      survey, 2–3, 9, 44
   anti-bullying policies, 151,
      see also Organisational
      culture change
   assessment of, 152–4
   definition of, 11–15, 116–17,
      151
   disapproval of, 122–4
   effects of, 76–101, 138
      case studies, 78–9
      costs, 79, 104, 150
      psychological effects, 20–1
      stress, 79–91
   gender differences, 18–23,
      67–8
   in midwifery education,
      91–101
      case studies, 93–4, 97
   of patients, 99–101

case studies, 99–100, 113
recognition of, 11, 16–18, 109
telltale signs, 130–1
within NHS, 1–5, 8–9, 11–12, 167
see also Aggression; Harassment

Change, management of, 141–7
Changing Childbirth, 26
Childhood experience, 45–7
case study, 46–7
Class difference, 32
Coaching, 152, 157
Codes of Practice, 108
Collaborative behaviour, 61–2
Communication, 41–2, 68–9
effects of male-dominated hierarchies, 41–2
Complaints procedure, 124–8
Concept-driven processing, 45
Constructive dismissal, 25
Coping strategies, 80, 137
Costs of bullying, 79, 104, 150
Counselling, 152
Criminal Justice and Public Order Act (1994), 104, 151
Cultural change, *see* Organisational culture change

Data-driven processing, 45
Destabilisation, 18
Disability Discrimination Act (1995), 105, 151
Dismissal, constructive, 25

Education, midwifery, 92

bullying in, 91–101
case studies, 93–4, 97
see also Training
Equal Opportunities Policy, 108
Existential neurosis, 80–1
Explicit personality theories, 64–5

First Contact scheme, 125

Gender issues, 59
attributional styles, 53
bullying styles, 18–23, 67–8
male-dominated hierarchies, 40–1
effects on women's communication, 41–2
Grievance procedure, 124–8
Groups, 62–3, 77, *see also* Teams

Halo effect, 51
Harassment, 11, 12, 15, 116, 125, 151
as criminal offence, 104–5, 150
see also Anti-harassment policy; Bullying; Sexual harassment
Health and Safety at Work Act (1974), 143, 151
Heresy factor, 59–61
Human Resource Management, 8–10, 38

I-A-B model for performance improvement, 119–21
Image, 50–1
Implicit personality theories, 49

Impression formation, 45, 48
  influencing factors, 49
  stereotyping, 49–52
Individual Performance Review
  (IPR), 119, 123
Information, dissemination of,
  128–9
Instrumental aggression, 66
Intimidating behaviour, 1, 58,
  88, 105–6, 166, *see also*
  Aggression; Bullying;
  Harassment
Isolation, 17

Jointism, 4

Kinship, 62–3

Language, 68–9
  body language, 69
Legislation, 104–12, 151
  case study, 106–7

Male-dominated hierarchies,
  40–1
  effects on women's
  communication, 41–2
Management culture, 37–8
Manufacturing Science and
  Finance union (MSF), 2, 8,
  14–15, 21
Mastery-drive theory, 59
Membership groups, 62–3
Mentoring schemes, 152
Midwifery education, 92
  bullying in, 91–101
  case studies, 93–4, 97
Midwifery Managers, 25, 26,
  88, 89, 167

Midwives, 30–1, 86
  bullying among, 1–3, 9,
  11–12, 22, 86–91
  case studies, 23–4, 86–7,
  90–1
  survey, 2–3, 9
  class difference, 32
  sociological factors, 32–7
  Supervisors, 22–3, 25, 86–8,
  98, 157
  support for, 157
Mobbing, 13

Negotiation skills, 154
Neuro-Linguistic Programming
  (NLP), 38, 70–1
NHS, 21
  bullying within, 1–5, 8–9,
  11–12, 167
  cultural change, 155, 156–7
  organisational purpose,
  155–6
  stress levels within, 81–5
Nurses, Midwives and Health
  Visitors Act (1979), 112
Nursing, 33–7

Observer fear, aggression and,
  142
Occupational health
  department, 141, 143
Organisational culture change,
  118–47
  case study, 145–6
  complaints procedure, 124–8
  disapproval of bullying,
  122–4
  dissemination of information,
  128–9

I-A-B model for performance improvement, 119–21
management of change, 141–7
NHS, 155, 156–7
organisational reputation, 141
shared values, 129–30
whistle blowing, 131–41
Overwork, 17–18

Patients, bullying of, 99–101
case studies, 99–100, 113
Peer pressure, 54–8
case study, 55–8
Perception, 45
influencing factors, 45–6
perceptual illusions, 47, 48
Performance:
I-A-B model for performance improvement, 119–21
Individual Performance Review (IPR), 119, 123
Personal standing, threat to, 17
Personality traits, 64–5
of bully, 65–6
of victim, 66–7
Post Traumatic Stress Disorder, 137
Power, 39–40
male-dominated hierarchies, 40–1
power profile, 63–4
Procedure, 41–2
Professional culture, 32–7
in management, 37–8
Professional status, threat to, 17
Projection, 51

Protection from Harassment Act (1997), 104–5, 151
Psychological effects of bullying, 20–1
Psychological theories, 44–5
attitudes, 54
attribution theory, 52–4
explicit personality theories, 64–5
impression formation, 48–9
Neuro-Linguistic Programming (NLP), 38, 70–1
peer pressure, 54–8
perception, 45–7
perceptual illusions, 48
stereotyping, 49–52
team psychology, 61–2
Psychometric testing, 38
Psychotic personality, 64–5
Public health movement, 30–1
Public Interest Disclosure Act (1999), 111–12, 135

Race Relations Act (1976), 105, 106, 151
Racism, 20, 27
Ramsay, Gordon, 19–20, 22
Recognition of bullying, 11, 16–18, 109
telltale signs, 130–1
Reference groups, 62–3
Risk assessment, 118
Risk management, 167
Royal College of Midwives (RCM), 2–3, 8
Equal Opportunities Policy, 108
survey, 2–3, 9, 44, 89, 94

Royal College of Nursing
(RCN), 8
Whistle Blow campaign,
132–4

Self-fulfilling prophecy, 51
Sex Discrimination Act (1975),
105, 106, 151
Sexual harassment, 19, 20, 27
attribution and, 53–4
see also Harassment
Shared values, 129–30
Sickness, 9, 83–4, 88–9, 130,
142–3, 150
Social learning theory, 58
Social reform, 30–1
Sociological factors, 32–7
Staff turnover, 21, 88–9, 150
Statutory Instruments (UKCC
1993), 112
Stereotyping, 49–52
Stress, 10, 76, 79–80, 89, 143
effects of, 79–91, 136–7
management of, 135–8,
152–4

within NHS, 81–5
workplace stressors, 76
Supervisors of Midwives, 22–3,
25, 86–8, 98, 157

Teams, 62–3, 84–5
team psychology, 61–2
Training, 128–9, 154–5
assertiveness, 154
see also Education,
midwifery
Transactional analysis, 71–3

Vicarious liability, 104
Victim culture, 8
Victims, 85
personality traits of, 66–7
procedure for, 158–63

Whistle blowing, 131–41
Public Interest Disclosure Act
(1999), 111–12, 135
Workplace bullying, *see*
Bullying
Workplace stressors, 76